Periodontal Instrumentation for the Practitioner

Periodontal Instrumentation for the Practitioner

Jill S. Nield-Gehrig, RDH, MA

Allied Health & Public Service Education
Asheville-Buncombe Technical Community College
Asheville, NC

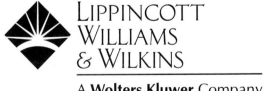

LIPPINCOTT
WILLIAMS
& WILKINS

A **Wolters Kluwer** Company

Editor: Larry McGrew
Project Editor: Ulita Lushnycky

Copyright © 1999 Williams & Wilkins
351 West Camden Street
Baltimore, Maryland 21201-2436 USA

Printed in the United States of America
First Edition, 1999

Library of Congress Cataloging-in-Publication Data
Nield-Gehrig, Jill S. (Jill Shiffer)
    Williams & Wilkins periodontal instrumentation for the
practitioner / Jill S. Nield-Gehrig.—1st ed.
        p.   cm.
    Includes bibliographical references and index.
    ISBN 0-683-30493-3
    1. Periodontics.   2. Periodontics—Instruments.   I. Title.
    [DNLM: 1. Periodontal Diseases—therapy.   2. Debridement—methods.
3. Periodontics—instrumentation.   WU 240 N667w 1999]
RK361.N54   1999
617.6′32—dc21
DNLM/DLC
for Library of Congress   98-21882
                                                                                CIP

The publishers have made every effort to trace the copyright holders for borrowed material. If they have inadvertently overlooked any, they will be pleased to make the necessary arrangements at the first opportunity.
To purchase additional copies of this book, call our customer service department at **(800) 638-0672** or fax orders to **(800) 447-8438.** For other book services, including chapter reprints and large quantity sales, ask for the Special Sales department. Canadian customers should call **(800) 665-1148,** or fax **(800) 665-0103.** For all other calls originating outside of the United States, please call **(410) 528-4223** or fax us at **(410) 528-8550.** *Visit Williams & Wilkins on the Internet:* http://www.wwilkins.com or contact our customer service department at **custserv@wwilkins.com.**

99 00 01 02 03
1 2 3 4 5 6 7 8 9 10

Preface

Williams & Wilkins "Periodontal Instrumentation for the Practitioner" is intended to provide dental health-care professionals with an update on current concepts in nonsurgical periodontal therapy. Present research findings challenge philosophic approaches that have served as the basis for clinical practice since the late 1960's. New treatment paradigms have emerged based on expanding knowledge of periodontal disease etiology coupled with new technologies. If clinicians are to continue to provide patients with the best possible care, they must incorporate current information into clinical practice.

New treatment paradigms and topics of growing concern to dental professionals are emphasized in this book. Chapter 1 contains information on work-related injuries such as, musculoskeletal disorders and latex hypersensitivity. Chapters 3, 4, 5, and 10 clarify current research findings and their application to periodontal debridement and extrinsic stain removal in daily practice. Chapter 6 addresses how technical advances in ultrasonic and sonic instrumentation can be used to enhance patient treatment.

This book is a concise and practical source of up-to-date treatment concepts. It is hoped that it will become a trusted reference for practicing dental healthcare professionals involved in providing nonsurgical therapy.

Jill S. Nield-Gehrig

Acknowledgments

The author would like to acknowledge the contributions of the following individuals; their help has been indispensable in bringing this book to completion.

Nancy Snyder Whitten, R.D.H, M.Ed., private practitioner, San Antonio, Texas, who reviewed the entire manuscript and made enormously helpful recommendations for its improvement

Rebecca Sroda, R.D.H., M.S., faculty, and John Dickson, computer information specialist, of Asheville-Buncombe Technical Community College for their contributions to the chapter on advanced fulcruming techniques

Charles D. Whitehead, the world's best medical illustrator, who created all the wonderful illustrations for the book

Dee Robert Gehrig, P.E., Gehrig Photographic Studio, and **Al J. Julian**—the talented individuals who created the many photographs for this book

The following individuals who were extremely generous with their time and knowledge: Beth Beathard, R.D.H, of EMS Electro Medical Systems; Mary Beth Lazzaro of Safeskin Corporation; Karen Neiner, R.D.H, B.S., of Hu-Friedy Manufacturing; and Noel E. Slotke, R.D.H., M.S., and Richard Paschke of DENTSPLY Preventive Care Division

Jill S. Nield-Gehrig

Contents

Registered Trademarks

The following are registered trademarks of:

American Eagle:
   EagleLite Suregrip instrument handle
   Gracey +3 Access Curettes
   Gracey +3 Deep Pocket Curettes

Branemark System Nobelpharma Implant Instruments

DENTSPLY Preventive Care:
   Cavitron ultrasonic scalers
   Cavitron JET with SPS Technology
   Cavitron SPS Ultrasonic Scaler with SPS
   Technology
   Dentsply BOBCAT ultrasonic scaler
   Steri-Mate sterilizable handpiece
   Midwest Quixonic sonic scaler
   SofTip disposable prophy tips
   Cavitron MED
   FSI Slimline (FSI-SLI) ultrasonic insert series
   Focused Spray (FSI) ultrasonic insert series
   Slimline (SLI) ultrasonic insert series
   Thru Flow (TFI) ultrasonic insert series
   DualSelect dispensing system
   Prophy-Jet 30
   JetShield aerosol reduction device for air polishing
   procedures

EMS (Electro Medical Systems):
   Piezon Master 400

ergoDent dental instrument grips

Ergodyne ProFles wrist supports

Florida Probe

Hu-Friedy:
    Slim-Flow ultrasonic inserts
    After Five instrument series
    Mini Five instrument series
    Vision Curvette instrument series
    Implacare plastic implant instruments

Impla-med Wiz-Stik implant instrument

Implant-Prophy+ implant instruments

Midwest:
    Quixonic Sonic Scaler
    SofTip disposable prophy tips

Premier:
    Periowise color-coded probe
    Premier implant scalers

SportsHealth Power Putty

Sultan Clearline microfiltration filter

Thompson Dental's Tactile Tone instrument handle

Titan sonic scaler

Welch Allyn WA DenLite illuminated dental mirror
Welch Allyn WA Reveal intraoral camera

Avoiding Work-Related Injuries

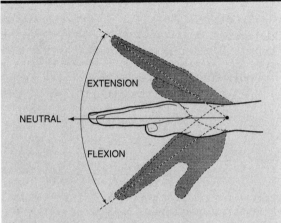

EXTENSION

NEUTRAL

FLEXION

In this chapter

Section 1:

Work-Related
Musculoskeletal Disorders

The National Institute for Occupational Safety & Health (NIOSH) defines a **work-related musculoskeletal disorder** as an injury affecting the musculoskeletal, peripheral nervous, and neurovascular systems that is caused or aggravated by occupational exposure to ergonomic hazards.

The dental health worker has a high risk of musculoskeletal injury when repetitive motions are combined with forceful movements, awkward postures, and insufficient recovery time.

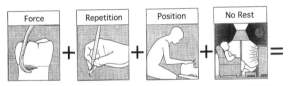

MUSCULOSKELETAL INJURY

According to the United States Bureau of Labor Statistics, musculoskeletal disorders result in more than 60% of all newly reported occupational injuries. Musculoskeletal disorders are experienced by computer operators, telephone operators, and bus drivers, as well as, dental healthcare workers. Treatments for musculoskeletal injuries include: rest, wrist splints, massage, anti-inflammatory medications, steroid injections, exercise, and surgery.

Musculoskeletal pain is a frequent symptom of practicing dentists, dental hygienists, and dental assistants. Occupational injuries to the muscles, nerves, and tendon sheaths of the back, shoulders, neck, arms, elbows, wrists, and hands are common among dental healthcare workers. Symptoms include loss of strength, tingling, numbness, and pain.

WORK-RELATED MUSCULOSKELETAL INJURIES	
Characteristics	• Develop gradually as a result of repeated microtrauma to an area • Have a slow onset • Are often ignored until the symptoms become chronic and permanent injury occurs
Activities Associated With Onset	• Ordinary movements such as gripping, twisting, and reaching • Activities become hazardous if they involve chronic repetition in a forceful and awkward manner with insufficient rest or recovery time
Predisposing Occupational Factors	• Repetitive movements of fingers, hand, and/or wrist • Awkward body positions • Static body position • Forceful pinching and/or gripping • Poorly fitting surgical gloves • Non-ergonomic equipment and instruments
Predisposing Health Conditions	• Diabetes • Gout • Rheumatoid arthritis • Hormonal changes (pregnancy, menopause, use of birth control pills) • Thyroid disorder • Alcoholism • Chronic renal disease • Stress • Collagen vascular disease

REPETITIVE MOTION

A repetitive motion is any motion that is repeated more than four times per minute. Anyone whose job involves forceful repetitive motions is at risk of a musculoskeletal injury. The human body was not designed to maintain the same body position or engage in repetitive movements for extended time periods. B.A. Silverstein, in an article in the British Journal of Industrial Medicine, defined a repetitive task as one that performs the same fundamental element for more than 50% of the cycle. A dental prophylaxis would certainly be categorized as a repetitive task under this definition. More than 50% of the time is spent performing very controlled, fast motions.

The Repetitive Nature of the Dental Hygiene Work-Cycle

The repetitive nature of the dental hygiene work-cycle was demonstrated in an ergonomic study commissioned by the Thompson Dental Supply Company. This study indicates that a typical work cycle for the dental hygienist is as follows: there are eight appointments on an average day, each appointment lasts an average of 45 minutes. Of the 45 minutes, approximately 30 minutes are used for debridement of tooth surfaces (scaling and root planing). The additional 15 minutes are used for other procedures and to provide education on home care. The dental hygiene work-cycle is depicted on page 6.

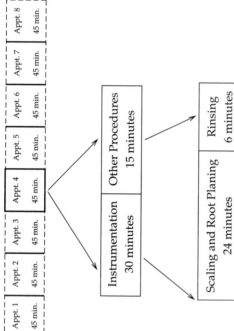

Reprinted with permission from Marley, R. et al, Thompson Dental Tool Study Final Report, University Technical Assistance Program, April 10, 1995.

Work Activity Assessment:
Risk Factor Identification Survey

Use this checklist to help you determine the presence of risk factors in your work setting. A "YES" answer indicates that changes are indicated in current work habits.

WORK CONDITION	YES	NO
1) Do you use frequent, repetitive motions?		
2) Do you perform the same motion or motion pattern every few seconds for more than a total of 2 to 4 hours?		
3) Does your postural work position include bending of the neck, shoulder, wrist, or finger joints?		
4) Do you maintain a fixed or awkward work posture (e.g., twisted or bent back) for 30 or more minutes?		
5) Do you make long reaches to obtain equipment or tools (greater than 18 inches from your body)?		
6) Do you make forceful or quick, sudden motions?		
7) Do you use forceful hand exertions for more than a total of 2 to 4 hours per day?		
8) Do you use a finger pinch grip?		
9) Do you maintain a fixed body position for extended time periods?		
10) Do you reach across the midline of your body or out to the side?		
11) Do you FAIL to adjust the height and location of equipment, chairs, and tools to provide for your personal size and comfort?		
12) Is the room temperature uncomfortable (too cold/too hot)?		

Adapted from (1) Proposed Occupational Safety and Health Administration (OSHA) Signal Risk Factors Form and (2) ErgoWeb ToolBox Risk Factor Identification Survey by ErgoWeb, Inc. (http://www.ergoweb.com).[2]

WORK-RELATED MUSCULOSKELETAL DISORDERS COMMONLY SEEN IN DENTAL HEALTHCARE WORKERS

Nerve Disorders

Carpal Tunnel Syndrome (CTS)

The carpal tunnel is a narrow channel in the wrist through which the vascular supply, flexor tendons, and median nerve cross into the hand from the arm. The flexor tendons can become inflamed from overuse; however, the carpal tunnel cannot expand in size to accommodate the increased mass of the inflamed tendons.

Symptoms: numbness, pain, and tingling in the thumb, index, and middle fingers

Causes:

1. Compression of the median nerve within the carpal tunnel of the wrist.
2. Compression in the neck and shoulder region—the nerve fibers that make up the median nerve originate in the spinal cord in the neck, therefore, poor posture can cause symptoms of CTS.

Ergonomic Hazards Resulting in CTS:

1. Upper body:
   • Poor posture in the neck and the upper chest
2. Wrist and hand:
   • Repeatedly extending the hand backward or downward
   • Repeatedly bending the wrist to either side
   • Pinch-gripping an instrument with excessive force or continuous pinch-grip without resting muscles

Areas of hand typically affected by symptoms of CTS.

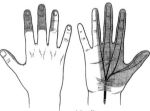

Median nerve

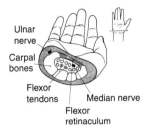
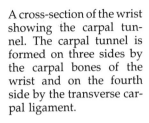

Ulnar nerve
Carpal bones
Flexor tendons
Median nerve
Flexor retinaculum

A cross-section of the wrist showing the carpal tunnel. The carpal tunnel is formed on three sides by the carpal bones of the wrist and on the fourth side by the transverse carpal ligament.

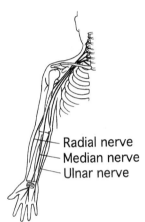

Radial nerve
Median nerve
Ulnar nerve

The radial, median, and ulnar nerves originate in the neck and terminate in the hand. The median nerve crosses into the hand within the carpal tunnel.

Ulnar Nerve Entrapment

The ulnar nerve supplies the muscles and skin on the ulnar side of the forearm and hand.

<u>Symptoms:</u> numbness, tingling, and loss of strength in the lower arm or wrist

<u>Causes:</u> Compression of the ulnar nerve of the arm as it passes through the wrist

<u>Ergonomic Hazards:</u>

- Repeatedly extending the hand backward or downward at the wrist

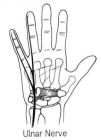

Ulnar Nerve

- Repeatedly bending the wrist to either side
- Holding the little finger a full span away from the hand

Pronator Syndrome

The pronator teres muscle is a superficial muscle of the forearm.

<u>Symptoms:</u> similar to symptoms of CTS

<u>Causes:</u> Compression of the median nerve between the two heads of the pronator teres muscle

<u>Ergonomic Hazard:</u> Holding the lower arm away from the body

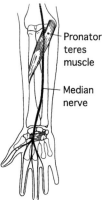

Pronator teres muscle

Median nerve

Tendon Disorders

Tendinitis of the Wrist

The tendons glide back and forth within a tendon sheath as the muscle contracts and relaxes. With overuse, the lubrication (synovial fluid) within the sheath becomes diminished.

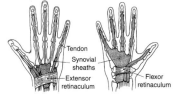

Tendon

Synovial sheaths

Extensor retinaculum

Flexor retinaculum

<u>Symptoms:</u> pain in the wrist, especially on the outer edges of the hand, rather than through the center of the wrist

<u>Causes:</u> inflammation of the tendons resulting from strain

<u>Ergonomic Hazard:</u> Repeatedly extending the hand backward or downward at the wrist

Tenosynovitis (De Quervain's Syndrome)

Affects the tendons on the side of the wrist and at the base of the thumb

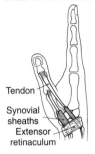

Tendon
Synovial sheaths
Extensor retinaculum

Symptoms: pain, especially on the side of the wrist and the base of the thumb; sometimes movement of the wrist yields a crackling noise over the tendon

Causes: Inflammation of the tendon sheath; overuse stimulates the production of excessive amounts of synovial fluid. This fluid accumulation results in a swollen, painful sheath.

Ergonomic Hazards:

- Hand twisting
- Forceful gripping
- Extending the hand backward or to the side

Rotator Cuff Tendinitis

Involves the muscle tendons in the shoulder region

Symptoms: severe pain and functional impairment of the shoulder

Causes: inflammation of the bursa (fluid-filled sac) that serves as a cushion for the muscle tendons as they slide back and forth over the rough bony surface of the humerus bone

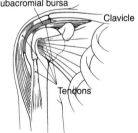

Subacromial bursa
Clavicle
Tendons

Ergonomic Hazards:

- Holding the elbow in an elevated position (above waist-level)
- Holding the upper arm away from the body

Muscular Disorder

Extensor Wad Strain

The extensor muscles serve to extend the fingers and thumb.

Symptoms: numbness, pain, and loss of strength in the fingers

Causes: injury to the extensor muscles of the thumb and fingers

Ergonomic Hazard: extending the fingers independently of each other

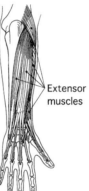

Extensor muscles

Neurovascular Disorders

Thoracic Outlet Syndrome

The thoracic outlet is an area at the base of the neck.

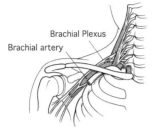

Brachial Plexus

Brachial artery

<u>Symptoms:</u> numbness, tingling, and/or pain in the fingers, hand, or wrist

<u>Causes:</u> compression of the brachial nerve plexus, the subclavian artery, and/or the subclavian vein between the neck and shoulder

<u>Ergonomic Hazards:</u>

- Tilting the head too far forward
- Hunching the shoulders forward
- Continuously reaching overhead

Surgical Glove-Induced Injury

Injury caused by improperly fitting gloves

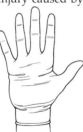

<u>Symptoms:</u> numbness, tingling, and/or pain in the wrist, hand, and/or fingers

<u>Causes:</u> improperly fitted surgical gloves

<u>Ergonomic Hazards:</u>

- Wearing gloves that are too tight across the palm of the hand and/or the wrist area
- Wearing ambidextrous gloves rather than right- and left-fitted gloves

Symptom Assessment

Use this checklist to help determine symptoms of a work-related musculoskeletal disorder. A "YES" answer to any question indicates that changes are needed in current work habits.*

SYMPTOMS	YES	NO
1) Do your hands or arms tingle or "burn"?	☐	☐
2) Do you experience tightness, discomfort, pain, or stiffness in your fingers, hands, wrists, forearms, or elbows?	☐	☐
3) Do you experience weakness in your hands or forearms?	☐	☐
4) Are you awakened at night with wrist pain or numb hands?	☐	☐
5) Do you feel the need to massage your hands, arms, or neck?	☐	☐
6) Do your hands fall asleep or feel abnormally cold?	☐	☐
7) Do you experience clumsiness or loss of strength and coordination in the hands?	☐	☐
8) Do you have difficulty using your fingers (e.g., buttoning clothing or putting on jewelry)?	☐	☐
9) Do you experience difficulty opening or closing your hands?	☐	☐
10) Do you experience pain in your neck, shoulders, upper back, or upper arms?	☐	☐
11) Do you have difficulty using your hands (e.g., writing, holding a coffee cup, turning door knobs, or opening or closing jars)?	☐	☐
12) Do you avoid activities or hobbies that you once enjoyed (e.g., needlepoint, knitting, tennis, golf)?	☐	☐

* This assessment is intended to introduce clinicians to the warning signs of work-related musculoskeletal disorders. Each disorder includes many more indicators than those presented here. *This assessment should not be used as the sole determinant of the presence or absence of work-related musculoskeletal disorders.* A complete assessment by a qualified physician is recommended.

Section 2:

Neutral Position for the Clinician

The **neutral position** is the ideal positioning of the body while performing work activities and is associated with decreased risk of injury. Poor body positioning is one of the major causes of musculoskeletal injury in dental healthcare workers. Research on musculoskeletal symptoms indicates that more than 80% of dental hygienists complain of pain in the upper body and back. It is generally believed that the more a joint deviates from the neutral position, the greater the risk of injury.

POSITIONS

The Neutral Seated Position

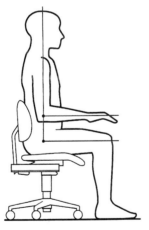

- Trunk and head erect
- Forearms and hands parallel to floor
- Weight evenly balanced
- Thighs parallel to the floor
- Seat height positioned low enough so that you are able to rest the heels of your feet on the floor
- Legs in a "V" formation, straddling the back of the patient chair when seated to the side or back of the patient

Your legs and the stool base should form a tripod, somewhat like the legs of a three-legged stool. This tripod formation creates a stable position from which to work.

AVOID: Positioning your legs together and under the back of the patient chair—this position requires you to raise your arms to reach the patient's mouth.

Neutral Neck Position

OK:

- Head tilt of 0° to 15°
- The line from your eyes to the treatment area should be as near to vertical as possible.

AVOID:

- Neck flexed at more than 20°

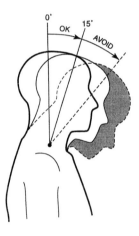

Neutral Shoulder Position

<u>OK:</u>

- Shoulders in horizontal line
- Muscles relaxed
- Weight evenly balanced when seated

<u>AVOID:</u>

- Lateral twisting of the head and neck
- Side-bending of the neck

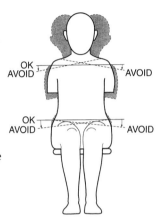

Neutral Back Position

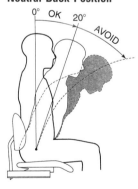

<u>OK:</u>

- Clinician may lean forward slightly <u>from the waist or hips.</u>
- Trunk flexion of 0° to 20°

<u>AVOID:</u>

- Overflexion of the spine (curved back)

Neutral Torso Position

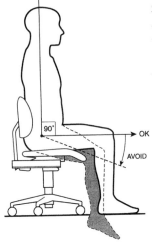

OK:

- Hip angle of 90°
- Weight evenly balanced on chair seat

AVOID:

- Trunk side-bending
- Weight not evenly balanced

Neutral Upper Arm Position

OK:

- Upper arms hang in a vertical line

AVOID:

- Upper arms lifted upward

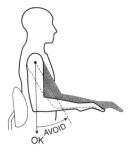

Neutral Upper Arm Position

<u>OK:</u>

- Elbows close to the sides of the body
- Abduction of elbows of 0° to 20° away from the body

<u>AVOID:</u>

- Upper arms held away from the body (abduction)
- Greater than 20° of abduction

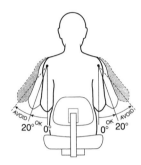

Neutral Forearm Position

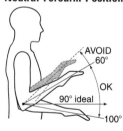

<u>OK:</u>

- Held parallel to the floor
- Raised, if necessary, by pivoting at the elbow joint

<u>AVOID:</u>

- Angle between forearms and upper arms of less than 60°.

Neutral Hand and Forearm Position

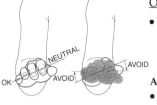

OK:

- Little finger–side of the hand and forearm is slightly lower than the thumb-side

AVOID:

- Pronation (i.e., rotating [turning] the forearm and hand inward, so that the thumb and little finger are level)

Neutral Wrist Position

OK:

- Wrist aligned with long axis of forearm

AVOID:

- Flexion (i.e., bending the wrist and hand down towards the palm)

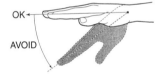

Neutral Wrist Position

OK:

- Wrist in alignment with forearm

AVOID:

- Extension (i.e., bending the wrist and hand up and back)

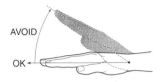

Neutral Wrist Position

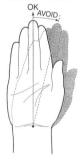

OK:

- Wrist aligned with long axis of forearm

AVOID:

- Radial deviation (i.e., bending the wrist toward the thumb)

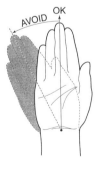

OK:

- Wrist aligned with long axis of forearm

AVOID:

- Ulnar deviation (i.e., bending the wrist toward the little finger)

WRIST DEVIATION TERMINOLOGY

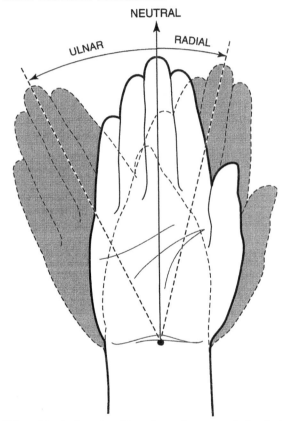

Ulnar Deviation: bending the wrist toward the little finger

Radial Deviation: bending the wrist toward the thumb

AN EASY TECHNIQUE: ESTABLISHING NEUTRAL POSITION IN RELATIONSHIP TO THE PATIENT

The most common ergonomic hazard is positioning the patient too high in relation to the clinician.

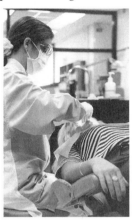

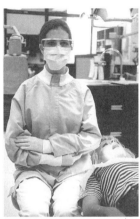

Incorrect positioning; patient too high.

Notice how the clinician must hold her arms up in a stressful position in order to reach the patient's mouth.

This error is often the result of a misconception that the clinician can see better if the patient is closer. Actually, the reverse is true; the clinician has improved vision of the mouth when the patient is in a lower position.

Determining the proper placement of the patient.

Sit alongside the patient with your arms against your sides and crossed at your waist. The patient's open mouth should be *below* the point of your elbow.

With the patient in this position, the clinician will be able to reach the mouth without placing stress on the muscles of her shoulders or arms.

THE ADJUSTABLE CLINICIAN CHAIR

The design of the clinician's chair should have the following characteristics

1. Legs—five legs for stability; casters for easy movement
2. Height
   - Height should allow clinician to sit with feet flat on floor and thighs parallel to the floor.
   - Height should be easily adjustable from a seated position; a seat height range of 14 to 20 inches will accommodate both tall and short clinicians.
3. Seat
   - Fabric that breathes (e.g., cloth rather than vinyl)
   - Front edge of seat should have a waterfall shape (rounded front edge).
   - Seat should not be too heavily padded; thick padding requires constant minor readjustments in order to maintain balance.
   - Seat length should allow clinician to sit with back against the backrest without impinging on the back of the knees. A seat length of 15 to 16 inches will fit most clinicians.
4. Backrest
   - Adjustable in vertical and horizontal positions so that it can be adjusted to support the lumbar region of the back when comfortably seated.
   - The angle between the seat and the chair back should be between 85 and 100°.

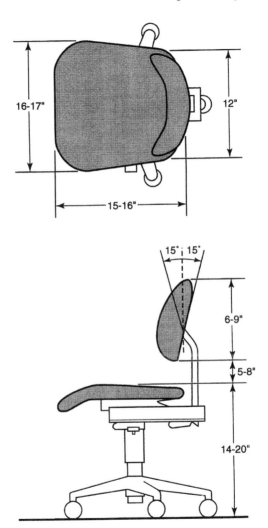

ERGONOMIC HAZARDS: CHANGING THOSE BAD HABITS!

The Tyranny of Subconscious Habits

As with any activity, it is easier to learn proper positioning from the start, rather than to change poor habits
once musculoskeletal injuries occur.

- Research shows that developed patterns of positioning physically alter the brain.
- It requires less effort and thought to engage an existing memory pattern for positioning.

The Process of Change

- Research by Dr. Gary Smith, Neuroscience, University of California, has shown that it takes 21 days
  to change a habit.
- To change a subconscious habit, you will have to
  stop and rethink the process each time that you begin it for at least 21 days.

MAKING A CHANGE

Suppose you decide to change the habit of raising your elbows above
waist-level when accessing the patient's mouth.—you will have to stop
and think about your positioning each time you access a treatment area
for *at least 21 days.*

Prevention of musculoskeletal injury requires a lifelong commitment to neutral positioning.

OPERATOR POSITIONING ZONES

The Right-Handed Clinician

Three positioning zones are used by the clinician. These
are the front, middle, and back positioning zones.

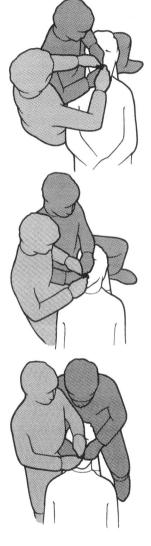

Front Zone, right-handed clinician.
The Front Zone extends from the front position to the side position.

Middle Zone, right-handed clinician.
The Middle Zone extends from the side position to the area adjacent to the temple region of the patient's head.

Back Zone, right-handed clinician.
The Back Zone extends from the area adjacent to the temple region of the patient's head to sitting directly behind the patient's head.

POSITIONING SUMMARY SHEET FOR THE RIGHT-HANDED CLINICIAN

Operator Positioning Zone	Treatment Area	Patient Position
Middle Zone (side to back position)	maxillary right posterior, lingual maxillary left posterior, facial	toward, chin-up toward, chin-up
Front Zone (front to side position)	maxillary right posterior, facial maxillary left posterior, lingual	straight, chin-up away, chin-up
Front Zone (front to side position)	maxillary anterior, surfaces toward	straight or turned slightly chin-up

Back Zone (back to directly behind)	maxillary anterior, surfaces away	straight or turned slightly chin-up
Middle Zone (side to back position)	mandibular right posterior, lingual mandibular left posterior, facial	toward, chin-down toward, chin-down
Front Zone (front to side position)	mandibular right posterior, facial mandibular left posterior, lingual	straight, chin-down away, chin-down
Front Zone (front to side position)	mandibular anterior, surfaces toward	straight, or turned slightly chin-down
Back Zone (back to directly behind)	mandibular anterior, surfaces away	straight, or turned slightly chin-down

The Left-Handed Clinician

Three positioning zones are used by the clinician. These are the front, middle, and back positioning zones.

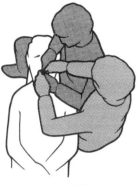

Front Zone, left-handed clinician:
The Front Zone extends from the front position to the side position.

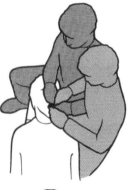

Middle Zone, left-handed clinician:
The Middle Zone extends from the side position to the area adjacent to the temple region of the patient's head.

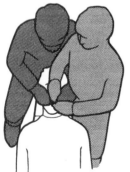

Back Zone, left-handed clinician:
The Back Zone extends from the area adjacent to the temple region of the patient's head to sitting directly behind the patient's head.

POSITIONING SUMMARY SHEET FOR THE LEFT-HANDED CLINICIAN

Operator Positioning Zone	Treatment Area	Patient Position
Middle Zone (side to back position)	maxillary right posterior, facial maxillary left posterior, lingual	toward, chin-up toward, chin-up
Front Zone (front to side position)	maxillary right posterior, lingual maxillary left posterior, facial	away, chin-up straight, chin-up
Front Zone (front to side position)	maxillary anterior, surfaces toward	straight or turned slightly chin-up
Back Zone (back to directly behind)	maxillary anterior, surfaces away	straight or turned slightly chin-up

continued

Operator Positioning Zone	Treatment Area	Patient Position
Front Zone (front to side position)	mandibular left posterior, facial mandibular right posterior, lingual	straight, chin-down away, chin-down
Middle Zone (side to back position)	mandibular left posterior, lingual mandibular right posterior, facial	toward, chin-down toward, chin-down
Front Zone (front to side position)	mandibular anterior, surfaces toward	straight, or turned slightly chin-down
Back Zone (back to directly behind)	mandibular anterior, surfaces away	straight, or turned slightly chin-down

Section 3:

Neutral Wrist Position During Instrumentation

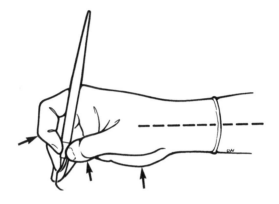

Neutral position of the wrist and fingers.

- Wrist aligned with long axis of lower arm.
- Little finger side of palm rotated slightly downward.
- Fingers held in rounded shape.
- Palm open and relaxed.

WRIST POSITION DURING INSTRUMENTATION

If you have a tendency to angle or bend your wrist and hand, a wrist brace can serve as a training tool to call your attention to wrist positioning. Inexpensive neoprene wrist braces are available in many pharmacies, sports stores, and business supply stores.

Ergonomic Hazard
The clinician in this photo is working with a bent wrist.

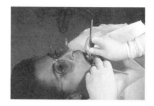

Failure to position the patient in a chin-down position forces the clinician to bend the wrist in order to position the instrument parallel to the long axis of the tooth.

Neutral Wrist Position
The clinician in this photo is working with the recommended neutral wrist position. The patient is correctly positioned in a full chin-down position.

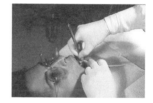

Carpal Tunnel Wrist Brace
If you are having a significant problem with neutral wrist position, you may want to train by using a carpal tunnel wrist brace. These specialized wrist braces are available at health supply stores and office supply companies. A lightweight, compact wrist support, the Proflex 4020 by Ergodyne, is shown.

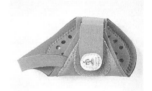

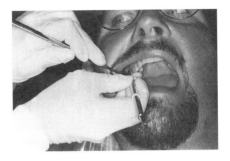

Ergonomic Hazard: The most common error in instrumenting the maxillary arch is resting the instrument handle against the knuckles of the index finger. With the handle in this position, the clinician must bend the wrist in order to align the handle with the long axis of the tooth.

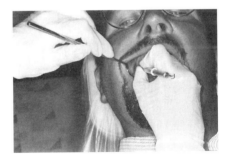

Neutral Wrist Position: The clinician in this photo is working with the recommended neutral wrist position. Wrist position is corrected by allowing the handle to rest in the "V" of the hand. This allows the clinician to establish parallelism without bending the wrist.

ARM AND WRIST MOTION FOR INSTRUMENT ACTIVATION

During stroke activation, the fingers, hand, wrist, and arm should be kept in a neutral position. The photograph shows the hand and arm when viewed from the side.

Use of the hand and arm is less fatiguing than using the fingers to provide the power for a calculus removal stroke.

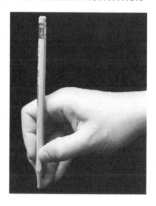

The movement is a rotating motion similar to the action of turning a door knob. Keeping the wrist in neutral position, from the ring finger fulcrum point, rotate the hand, wrist, and forearm as a unit.

The photograph shows the hand and arm when viewed from behind.

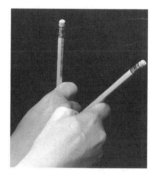

Mechanics check during an instrument stroke: The hand, wrist, and arm move as a *single unit* to produce the motion for each instrumentation stroke. Maintain the wrist in neutral position during motion activation.

SUMMARY: NEUTRAL POSITION FOR THE CLINICIAN

Structure	Correct Body Mechanics	Incorrect Body Mechanics
Head	• Erect, neck aligned with torso	• Tilted to one side • Tipped too far forward
Shoulders	• Relaxed, aligned with torso	• Lifted up toward ears • Tense • Hunched forward
Upper Arms	• Held slightly away from body	• Raised above waist level
Elbows	• At waist level, slightly away from body	• Raised above waist level
Wrist	• Aligned with lower arm • Little finger–side of palm is slightly lower than thumb-side of palm	• Palm and wrist bent upward • Hand and wrist bent downward • Hand angled toward body • Hand angled away from body • Thumb-side of palm rotated down so that palm is parallel to floor

continued

Structure	Correct Body Mechanics	Incorrect Body Mechanics
Fingers and Hand	• Correct glove size • Fingers relaxed in grasp	• Gloves too tight • Excessive finger pressure against handle • Fingers tense
Back	• Straight, may bend forward slightly from the waist or hips	• Rounded back
Hips	• Back on seat • Body balanced on seat • Weight evenly distributed	• Perched forward on seat • All weight on one hip or the other
Legs	• Parallel to floor or knees slightly higher than hips • Straddle the patient chair back when seated to side of the back of patient	• Legs under the patient chair back • Leaning all weight on one leg or the other • Knees lower than hips • Thighs "cut" by edge of chair seat • Legs crossed
Feet	• Stool positioned so that you can place your heels flat on the floor • Feet spread apart so your legs and the chair base form a tripod-shaped base.	• Feet dangling • Ankles crossed • Foot or feet resting off floor, such as on chair rail or caster

Section 4:

Instrument Handles

Recommended:	Avoid:
• Large diameter handles • 3/8-inch in diameter • Light-weight handles • Highly textured handles	• Small diameter handles • 3/16-inch in diameter • Solid metal handles • Smooth or finely textured handles

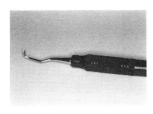

The EagleLite Suregrip handle from American Eagle Instruments is 50% larger in diameter and 26% lighter in weight than traditional instrument handles.

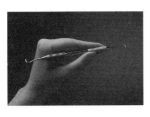

The Tactile Tone handle from Thompson Dental has medical-grade silicone sleeves. The silicone sleeves spread the pressure of the grasp over the entire finger pad.

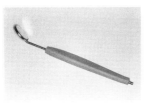

ErgoDent mirror handles from The Nordic Group, Inc., are made of a rubberlike plastic that provides a soft and secure hold. The mirror handle is triangular in cross-section and is autoclavable.

Section 5:

Gloves and
Glove-Associated Reactions

GLOVES: MAINTAINING EFFECTIVE BARRIER PROTECTION

To optimize protection, dental healthcare workers should understand proper glove selection, storage, and use.

Issues	Recommendations
Glove Type	1. Latex—provide the most durable barrier protection; good flexibility 2. Nitrile—provide good dexterity and is tougher than latex 3. Neoprene, Polymer, PVC—much less durable than latex 4. Vinyl—least durable; not flexible, breaks rather than gives
Glove Storage	• Store boxes in a cool, dry, dark area with good ventilation • Avoid exposure to intense light, prolonged heat, or excessive moisture • Store away from direct light (sunlight or artificial) • Store away from electrical equipment such as ultrasonic units, radiograph machines, or generators
Hands	• Maintain high level of hand care; cracks in skin provide access for bacterial, viral, and fungal invasion • Rinse hands thoroughly after washing or exposure to disinfectants; soaps and disinfectants are common skin irritants

continued

Issues	Recommendations
	• Maintain short fingernails to prevent punctures • During non-work hours, apply hand lotions to maintain skin integrity
Hand Lotions	Avoid use of lotions or medications (e.g., petroleum-based lotions or those containing lanolin, cocoa butter, mineral oil, or jojoba oil) under gloves that can compromise the integrity of latex or synthetic glove material
Jewelry	Remove jewelry before donning gloves: • Jewelry presents a puncture hazard • Jewelry interferes with thorough washing and rinsing of hands and increases the risk of skin irritation
Glove Size	• Select fitted gloves (right- and left-handed) • If you are experiencing symptoms of musculoskeletal injury involving your hands, use right- and left-hand fitted gloves that come in a full range of sizes (i.e.: 5½, 6, 6½, 7, 7½, etc., rather than S, M, L) • Gloves come in a wide variety of configurations (e.g., rounded or tapered fingers, narrow or broad palms). Ask your supplier for samples. • Select gloves of the correct size or a little loose. Gloves should never be tight across the palm or at the wrist.
Glove Use	Change gloves every hour: • The probability of puncturing the glove material increases over time • Gloves are non-ventilating, except at the cuffs • If hands are sweaty or the skin is wrinkled, then the gloves have been on too long. Wash and rinse hands thoroughly in-between glove changes.

PROPER FIT FOR SURGICAL GLOVES

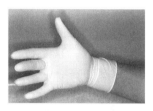

Avoid

- Gloves that are tight-fitting across the wrist and/or palm of the hand.

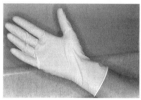

Recommended
The index finger of your opposite hand should slip easily under the wrist area of the gloved hand. Select gloves with textured surfaces for improved grip.

GLOVE-ASSOCIATED REACTIONS: LATEX ALLERGY

Since 1980, healthcare workers have been exposed to more and more latex, especially in the form of disposable latex gloves. As a result of universal precautions for infection control, healthcare professionals are using gloves more often and changing them more frequently. The dental community has become increasingly concerned about the effects of using materials that contain latex for personnel and patients who are latex-sensitive. By September 1992, 1,100 reactions and 15 fatalities related to latex allergy had been reported to the Food and Drug Administration (FDA), prompting them to issue a Medical Alert to healthcare professions. The FDA estimates that less than 1% of the general population has latex sensitivity. Estimates for healthcare workers are much higher, from 3 to 12%, depending on the study. People with spina bifida, who were continually exposed to latex tips on enema bottles as children, are at the highest risk. The FDA estimates that up to 68% of people with this birth defect are latex sensitive.

Because of the nature of the profession, dental professionals commonly wear gloves 8 to 10 hours daily, up to five days per week. This increased exposure has been cited as the probable cause for the high prevalence of latex sensitivity in the dental profession. The infection control guidelines of all major Dental Associations now recommend that dental healthcare professionals wear protective gloves for all treatment procedures. It is possible, therefore, that recent dental and dental hygiene graduates face 40 years of glove-wearing.

Latex is the natural sap of the rubber tree, *Hevea braziliensis*. Natural rubber latex (NRL) is used in the production of 40,000 industrial products used in the United States. Many patients erroneously believe they are allergic to the powder used on latex gloves. Starch powders actually are rare allergens, but they do act to absorb the latex proteins and chemicals and carry them airborne. Substances such as chemicals, endotoxins, silicone, and biocides bind to the powder particles during the manufacturing process of sterile and non-sterile gloves. Latex products contain two types of compounds that cause medical problems, (1) added chemicals such as accelerators, which cause dermatitis, and (2) natural proteins, which cause systemic potentially life-threatening immediate allergic reactions in the sensitized individual.

TERMINOLOGY

NRL is the natural rubber latex derived from the natural sap of the rubber tree, *Hevea braziliensis*.

Well-processed powdered gloves should have protein levels at or below 150 micrograms per gram (μg/g). Powdered gloves that are not well-processed may have powder levels more than 2,500 μg/g.

Well-processed, powder-free gloves should have protein levels at or below 50 μg/g.

Hypoallergenic indicates less likely to cause irritant contact dermatitis or allergic contact dermatitis. A label of "hypoallergenic" does not mean that a product is latex-free.

Chemical contact sensitizers are specific chemicals found in gloves that trigger a cell-mediated allergic response in certain patients.

Aerosolized latex protein allergens are the protein allergens bound to cornstarch powder particles, which then become airborne. This aerosolized "latex dust" can remain airborne for up to 12 hours in ambient circulating air. Hundreds of thousands of these contaminated powder particles are launched into the air during the donning, "snapping," or removal of powdered gloves.

Touch contamination is the transfer of microorganisms and chemicals adhering to powder particles on powdered gloves to the healthcare worker and the patient. Transfer of contaminated powder particles may occur through direct touch or through inhalation of airborne powder particles.

Anaphylactic Shock is the most severe form of allergic reaction that produces respiratory distress and airway obstruction. It is a life-threatening medical emergency; airway obstruction from laryngeal edema or cardiovascular collapse from vasodilation may lead to death at any moment. Hoarseness or stridor are signs of laryngeal edema and indicate the possibility of impending airway obstruction.

WHO IS AT RISK? PREDISPOSING CONDITIONS:

1. Individuals who had multiple surgeries early in life
2. Individuals with a history of recurrent surgical procedures or multiple hospitalizations
3. Individuals who frequently wear latex gloves (i.e., dental healthcare providers, medical operating room personnel)
4. Individuals with a history of hay fever, asthma, multiple drug allergies, or hay fever
5. Individuals with a history of allergy to any of the following foods: avocado, apple, pear, celery, carrot, hazelnut, kiwi, papaya, pineapple, peach, cherry, plum, apricot, banana, melon, chestnut, nectarine, grape, fig, passion fruit, tomatoes, and/or potatoes
6. Individuals with eczema
7. Individuals with spina bifida—the prevalence of latex allergy has been reported to be as high as 68%. For this reason, all patients with spina bifida should be regarded as latex sensitive.
8. Individuals with a history of repeated bladder catheterization; these include patients with neural tube defects (i.e., myelomeningocele/ meningocele, spina bifida), spinal cord trauma, urogenital malformations, and neurogenic bladder.
9. Individuals with hand dermatitis that is severe or has changed in severity

Note: Severe allergic reactions in patients with NO apparent risk factor are rare but have been documented.

Latex-sensitive individuals should be advised to wear proper identification, such as a Medic Alert bracelet that warns of their latex allergy. Individuals who have experienced allergic contact dermatitis or immediate allergic reactions should carry their own epinephrine auto-injector, such as EpiPen (Center Laboratories, Port Washington, NY) or Ana Kit (Bayer Corporation Pharmaceutical Division, West Haven, CT).

THREE TYPES OF GLOVE-ASSOCIATED REACTIONS

Photographs courtesy of Safeskin Corporation.

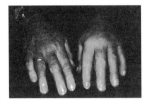

1. Irritant Contact Dermatitis: dermatitis caused by chemical irritation that does not involve the immune system

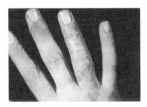

2. Allergic Contact Dermatitis: a contact dermatitis caused by chemicals used in glove production but involving the immune system

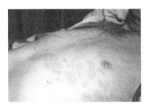

3. Immediate Allergic Reaction: an allergic reaction caused by latex proteins; this type can result in serious and potentially fatal reactions.

Irritant Contact Dermatitis is a non-allergic skin rash that does not involve the immune system. Irritant contact dermatitis can result from wearing either latex or synthetic gloves. It is a non-life threatening condition.

Also known as	Non-allergic dermatitis
Symptoms	Dry thickened skin, cracking, and sores; symptoms may be worse on knuckles, wrist, and back of the hand
Extent	Stops at glove boundary
Susceptibility	Anyone can experience
Causes	1. Skin irritation from non-glove–related substances such as soaps, detergents, or disinfectants, especially if left on the skin after insufficient hand rinsing 2. Jewelry unnecessarily increases the potential for irritation by inhibiting proper hand rinsing. 3. The drying effect of glove powder 4. Skin irritation from chemical additives from the glove manufacturing process 5. Irritation from sweating under the gloves—perspiration trapped against the skin by the glove is absorbed into the cells, which become hyperhydrated and fragile, increasing the possibility of irritation.
Prevention of skin irritation	• Remove jewelry. • Wash hands with a mild soap each time gloves are removed, and rinse thoroughly. • Change gloves frequently. • Wear a larger size glove to increase air circulation to skin. • During off-duty hours, use a hand lotion.
If you experience this reaction	1. Switch glove brands. 2. Use cotton, PVC, or polyethylene liners. The glove liner should be changed each time that gloves are changed. Cotton liners can be laundered and reused. 3. See a dermatologist.

Allergic Contact Dermatitis is a skin rash caused by a cell-mediated allergic response activated by repeated contact with the allergen. Chemicals added in the glove manufacturing process of synthetic and latex gloves are the most frequent causes of allergic contact dermatitis.

Also known as	Type IV Dermatitis and Delayed Type Hypersensitivity
Symptoms	Acute: small clustered vesicles that are painful when scratched Chronic: dry, red, cracking, crusted, and thickened skin with hard bumps, sores, and sometimes blisters
Extent	May extend up the arm beyond glove boundary
Susceptibility	History of allergy is a predisposing factor.
Causes	1. Chemical additives implicated in allergic contact dermatitis include accelerators, antioxidants, anti-microbials, emulsifiers, dispersing agents, colorants, and stiffeners. 2. Accelerators are the most common cause of glove-related allergic contact dermatitis. Different accelerators (e.g., thiurams, carbamates, mercaptobenzothiazole [MBT]) are used by various glove manufacturers.
Reduce risk of sensitization to chemical additives	Select a glove documented low in chemical additives.
If you experience this reaction	1. See a dermatologist. 2. Select a glove with a different accelerator. If condition does not improve, isolate the specific allergen (i.e., accelerator, antioxidant, colorant, biocide, or preservative).

Immediate Allergic Reaction is an allergic reaction caused by protein antibodies in the latex. This type can result in serious and potentially life-threatening reactions.	
Also known as	Systemic Reaction, Immediate Hypersensitivity Reaction, Urticaria, and Protein Allergy
Symptoms	Hives, facial swelling, watery eyes, itchy eyes, inflamed eyes, eyelid swelling, runny nose, difficulty breathing, pharyngeal swelling, abdominal cramps, dizziness, low blood pressure, rapid heart beat, and anaphylactic shock
Extent	May involve any part of the body
Susceptibility	• Patients with spina bifida should be treated as if they are latex sensitive. • Healthcare workers • Patients with a history of allergy • Patients with a history of food allergies to one or more of the following: bananas, avocados, chestnuts, kiwis, papaya, fig, nectarine, plum, passion fruit, tomatoes, cherries, melons, celery, and potatoes.

Causes	1. An IgE-mediated response to latex proteins
	2. Routes of exposure to the latex proteins include:
	  • direct contact with dermal or mucosal surfaces,
	  • inhalation of aerosolized latex protein allergens, and
	  • direct contact during invasive procedures, such as surgical or extraction procedures.
	3. Individuals who experience allergic contact dermatitis may be predisposed by constant sensitization over time to develop into an immediate allergic reaction.

continued

Reduce risk of sensitization	Select a powder-free glove that is low in latex protein.
If you experience this reaction	1. Select a non-latex (synthetic) glove. 2. Coworkers in the dental office should wear powder-free latex gloves to prevent production of aerosolized powder. 3. See an allergist. 4. Carry EPI-Pen in case of anaphylactic reaction.

GLOVE POWDER HAZARDS IN THE DENTAL OFFICE	
Processing	Potential powder transference from gloves to instruments and equipment during processing
Treatment Room	• Wound contamination with glove powders during surgical or extraction procedures ⇒ acute inflammation of wound site ⇒ delayed wound healing ⇒ increased risk of infection • Inhaled aerosolized powder risk for healthcare worker and patient ⇒ immediate allergic reaction to airborne latex protein allergens • Allergic contact dermatitis to bound glove chemicals
Employee Health	• Hands: ⇒ lipid absorption ⇒ skin abrasion ⇒ contact dermatitis (irritant or allergic) ⇒ Type I hypersensitivity to latex protein allergens ⇒ breach of the skin's protective barrier • Lungs: ⇒ immediate allergic reaction to powder-transported latex protein allergens ⇒ irritant asthma trigger • Migration of contaminated powder can cause: ⇒ clogged or infected sinuses ⇒ inflammation or infection of the middle ear
Immune Compromised Patient	• Potential contamination of opportunistic natural flora from healthcare worker or patient • Pathogenic microorganisms carried on powder may result in severe infection • Powder on non-sterile gloves may sustain microorganisms, which may be inhaled

Adapted from ''Guide For Managing Powder In The Healthcare Environment,'' Safeskin Corporation Education Series, 1994.

SAMPLE LATEX ALLERGY SCREENING QUESTIONNAIRE

1. Are you a healthcare worker?

2. Do you wear latex gloves regularly or are you otherwise exposed to latex regularly?

3. Do your fellow workers wear latex or rubber gloves regularly?

4. Have you ever been tested for allergies? If yes, what were the results?

5. Do you have hay fever, asthma, or other allergies?

6. Do you have a history of anaphylaxis (i.e., swelling of the throat, difficulty breathing)?

7. Have you experienced eczema or rashes on your hands?

8. Do you have or think that you have an allergy to latex rubber?

9. Circle any foods below that cause hives, itching of the lips or throat, or other symptoms when you eat or handle them:
   avocado, apple, pear, celery, carrot, hazelnut, kiwi, papaya, pineapple, peach, cherry, plum, apricot, banana, melon, chestnut, nectarine, grape, fig, passion fruit, tomatoes, or potatoes

10. Do the following swell or itch when you have dental work done: your face, lips, or tongue?

11. Have you had a tingling or burning sensation during dental treatment?

12. How many surgeries, including dental, have you had? Did any of these take place when you were an infant?

13. Have you had itching, swelling, or other symptoms following dental, rectal, or pelvic exams?

14. Do your hands break out when you use rubber gloves?

15. Have you experienced swelling or difficulty breathing after blowing up a balloon?

16. Do rubber handles, rubber bands, or elastic bands on clothing cause any discomfort?

MANAGEMENT OF THE LATEX-SENSITIVE PATIENT

When caring for a patient with a known or suspected latex allergy:

1. Clearly indicate the allergy on the patient's chart.
2. Instruments used in the patient's treatment must not have been handled, at any point, by an individual wearing latex gloves. For example, latex gloves should not be worn when instruments are placed in autoclave bags or instrument trays for sterilization. Latex remains on the instruments throughout the sterilization process. As a general rule, it is good practice to wear non-latex gloves during the processing (e.g., scrubbing, bagging) of instruments.
3. Thoroughly assess the treatment room to minimize any latex exposure.
4. All healthcare workers who will come in direct contact with the patient should wear non-latex gloves. Personnel who will be handling <u>instruments or other items</u> to be used during treatment of the patient should wear non-latex gloves.
5. Take an adequate patient history before performing dental treatment.

TREATMENT FOR SEVERE ALLERGIC REACTION

1. Call 911.
2. Epinephrine 1:1000, 0.3 cc subcutaneously stat (children 1:1000, 0.01 ml/kg up to 30 kg)
3. Salbutamol 2 puffs (if patient conscious and wheezy)
4. Place patient in a head down position (Trendelenburg).
5. Administer oxygen by nasal cannula.
6. Do not leave patient.
7. Ensure patient airway.
8. Monitor vital signs.
9. Initiate cardiopulmonary resuscitation if required.
10. Until the patient is transferred to emergency medical personnel, repeat epinephrine every 10 minutes if the patient is experiencing significant symptoms indicating a need for further epinephrine.

Latex Containing Materials Commonly Used in a Dental Office

Please Note: Products are constantly changing. <u>Check with suppliers before using any product with a latex-allergic individual.</u> Companies listed under "Alternatives" also make many latex products; usually only selected products in a company's product line are latex-free.

Materials	Sources of Latex Safe Alternatives
Ambu Bag	Armstrong Medical - (800) 323-4220 Laerdal - (800) 431-1055 Nellcor Puritan-Bennet - (800)-NELLCOR Respironics - (800) 345-6443 Pacific Rim Dental - (800) 298-9074
Attire	Disposable gowns and masks may contain latex and the finish may have irritants to a latex-sensitive person. Wear reusable gowns.
Band-Aids	3M Active Strips Snippy Brand - Quantasia Readi-Bandages or use sterile gauze with plastic tape
Bite Block	Patterson Dental Supply Co.
Blood pressure cuff and tubing	Use over patient's clothing Critikon - (813) 887-2000 (Dinamap) PyMaH - (800) 526-3538 (Perfect Balance) Vital Signs - (800) 932-0760 (Cleen Cuff)
Dental Dam Material	The Hygienic Corporation SmartPractice - (800) 522-0800 Hager Worldwide - (800) 328-2335 (silicone dam material)
Dental Gutta Percha	ESPE-Premier Ketac Endo

continued

Materials	Sources of Latex Safe Alternatives
Denture Resin	Astron Dental Corp. - Ultimate 1180 vinyl denture resin
Ice Wraps	Propac 11 (Carolon)
Endotracheal Tubes, airways	Bermain - (617) 737-7855 Mallinckrodt - (800) 262-3654 Polemedco Airways - (310) 577-1422
Gloves, surgical and exam	Allerderm Laboratories - (800) 365-6868 Ansell Medical - (800) 524-1377 Ansell/Perry - (800) 321-9752 Baxter Health Care Corporation - (800)-4-BAXTER Best Manufacturing - (800) 241-0323, (800) 819-6980 ECI Medical, Nova Scotia, Canada - 800-NOT-LATEX Hermal Pharmaceutical - (800) 437-6251 Johnson & Johnson - (800) 526-3967 Maxxim - (800) 727-7340 Medline Catalog - 1-800-MEDLINE Regent Medical - (800) 843-8494 Safeskin Corporation - (800) 462-9989 Smart Practice - (800) 522-0800
Impression Materials	Alginate impression materials do not contain rubber
Local Anesthetic Carpules (stoppers in the pre-filled carpules and the diaphragm at top of the cartridge contains latex)	Wyeth

continued

Materials	Sources of Latex Safe Alternatives
Masks, Face	Alternative Resource Catalog - (800) 618-3129 Biotrol - (800) 822-8550 Kimberly Clark - (800) 524-3577 SmartPractice - (800) 522-0800 Sultan - (800) 637-8582 Technol, Inc. - (800) 433-4026 x6485
Nitrous Oxide Equipment	Accutron, Inc. SmartPractice - (800) 522-0800
Orthodontic Bands	Midwest Orthodontic Manufacturing and Maser Industries
Prophy Cups/ Angles	John O. Butler Company SmartPractice - (800) 522-0800
Stethoscope tubing	Armstrong Medical - (800) 323-4220 Cover with ScopeCoat - (800) 373-0747
Syringes, disposable (stoppers contain latex)	Air-Tite - (800) 257-5318; suppliers of HSW, Air-Tite, Terumo, and B-D syringes. Terumo Medical Corporation - (800) 862-4882 Or if latex-free syringe is not available, draw up medication in syringe right before use and administer immediately
Syringes, auto injectable	Epi-Pen by Center Labs - (800) 223-6837
Utility gloves (kitchen gloves)	Magla - PVC Myplex Allerderm -cotton liners - (800) 365-6868 Williams and Sonoma - household nitrile - (800) 541-2233
Resource Catalog	Medline's Latex Free Catalog - more than 1,000 products including surgical gloves - 1-800-MEDLINE

Latex Allergy Resources

Information about latex allergy is available from these resources:

1. A.L.E.R.T., Inc. (Allergy to Latex Education and Resource Team)
   P.O. Box 23722, Milwaukee, WI 53223 Telephone: (888) 97ALERT
   Internet   address: http://www.execpc.com/~trukaras/ALERT
2. ELASTIC (Education for Latex Allergy/Support Team & Information Coalition)
   196 Pheasant Run Road, West Chester, PA 19380 Telephone: (610) 436-4801
3. Latex Allergy Support Links internet site: http://pw2.netcom.com/~nam1/latexallergy.html

---

LATEX EXPOSURE GUIDELINES

1. Review use of latex gloves for various tasks. Determine if latex gloves are appropriate for the level of protection and degree of risk. Recommend use of non-latex gloves where appropriate.

2. Use powder-free, low protein gloves whenever possible to reduce direct skin exposure and exposure to airborne latex proteins. Check with the manufacturer to be certain that gloves to be purchased have low protein levels and low levels of chemical sensitizers.

3. Identify workers who are at risk. Train staff about potential health risks to healthcare workers and patients.

4. Care must be taken to ensure that filtration and ventilation systems provide adequate fresh air. Clean filtration and ventilation systems thoroughly on a regular basis.

5. Promote relevant patient education about latex allergy.

6. Identify patients at risk. Establish procedures for providing treatment in a latex safe environment.

7. Assure the availability of prompt, appropriate emergency treatment, should an allergic reaction occur. The dental team should be fully trained in emergency management of anaphylactic shock.

Section 6:

Additional Strategies for Avoiding Injury

STRATEGIES DURING INSTRUMENTATION

The very nature of periodontal debridement means that the clinician uses repetitive movements during instrumentation. One of the most damaging aspects of repetitive movements is the result of maintaining the muscles in the same position for extended time periods. You can reduce muscle strain in several ways as you work.

1. **RELAX.** Only apply muscle pressure *during* a work stroke for calculus removal or root surface debridement. Keep the muscles of your fingers, hand, and wrist relaxed at all other times.
2. **SLOW DOWN.** Strokes should <u>not</u> be made in a rapid, non-stop manner. Remember that the faster the pace of your strokes, the more difficult it is to control them. Slow down, take your time making each stroke, and pause between strokes. Your strokes will be more accurate, and your muscles will be more relaxed.
3. **PAUSE.** Pause at the end of each stroke to relax your muscles. This does not mean that you should take your hand out of the mouth and lay the instrument down every time that you make a stroke. It means that you relax your muscles so that you are lightly grasping the instrument handle in the mouth. Your muscles should remain relaxed as you reposition the working end in preparation for your next stroke. In terms of avoiding a musculoskeletal injury, this step is the most important step that you can take.
4. **DIGITAL ACTIVATION.** Give your wrist and arm muscles a rest by using digital motion activation when appropriate. Digital activation is indicated for: 1) exploring and probing, 2) instrumenting furcations, and 3) using ultrasonic or sonic instruments.

5. **PATIENT SCHEDULING.** Avoid scheduling two patient cases in a row that are instrumentation-intensive. Try to alternate cases that are instrumentation-intensive with easier cases or activities such as a full mouth radiograph series. Schedule instrumentation-intensive cases early in the day.

Short Work Breaks

Stretches

You will need little recovery time between instrumentation-intensive activities to cool and lubricate muscles and tendons. A 10 minute break each hour from instrumentation provides sufficient recovery time. Without short breaks, the need for recovery builds and the threat of injury increases.

> **Caution:** As with any exercise, do not do any stretch if it hurts. If you have or suspect that you may have a musculoskeletal disorder, do not attempt these stretches without the permission of a physician.

1. **During Instrumentation.** Approximately every 20 minutes, stop and return the instrument to your tray set-up. Stretch your fingers apart, and hold the stretch for a few seconds. Relax your muscles, and slowly curl your fingers inward without clenching. Keep your fingers curled for a few seconds before repeating. Repeat several times. As with any exercise, do not do this if it hurts!
2. **During instrumentation or between patients.** Rest your eyes periodically by focusing on distant objects.
3. **During instrumentation or between patients.** Drop your hands to your sides and shake them gently as though you were trying to shake off drops of water. This improves blood circulation. As with any exercise, do not do this if it hurts!
4. **Between Patients.** Hold a soft foam ball in your hand with your palm up. Maintaining a palm up

position, gently squeeze the ball five to ten times. Repeat with the opposite hand. As with any exercise, do not do this if it hurts!

5. **Between Patients.** Rub the palms of your hands together until they feel warm. Close your eyes, and cup your warmed hands over them. Relax and concentrate on your breathing as you slowly exhale and inhale for 5 to 10 seconds.

Relaxation Stretches Between Patients

These stretches should be done slowly and deliberately, allowing for complete relaxation after each repetition. Breathe deeply during all of the stretches.

> **Caution:** As with any exercise, do not do any stretch if it hurts. If you have or suspect that you may have a musculoskeletal disorder, do not attempt these stretches without the permission of a physician.

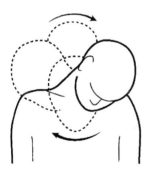

Head Rolls:
To relax the neck and shoulder muscles

1. Stand or sit. Concentrate on your breathing as you do this stretch.
2. Exhale, and slowly roll your head to the right. Inhale deeply.
3. Exhale, and slowly roll your head to the left. Inhale deeply.
4. Exhale, and lower your chin to your chest. Inhale deeply, and raise your chin.
5. Repeat steps going in the opposite direction.

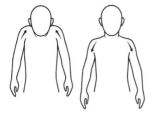

Shoulder Shrugs:
To relax shoulder and up-
per back muscles

1. Stand or sit.
2. Inhale, and slowly
   pull your shoulders
   up toward your ears.
   Hold for 10 seconds.
3. Exhale, and slowly
   lower your shoulders
   to a relaxed position.
4. Repeat.

Shoulder Rolls:
To relax shoulder and up-
per back muscles

1. Stand or sit.
2. Pull your shoulders
   back, then up, then
   forward, then down in
   a circular motion.
3. Roll 5 times forward,
   then 5 times back-
   ward.

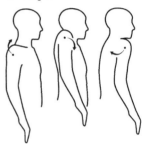

Side Bends:
To stretch the muscles of
the trunk and upper back

1. Sit.
2. Interlace your fingers,
   and lift your arms up
   over your head.
3. Press your arms back-
   ward as far as you can.
4. Exhale, and slowly
   lean to one side. In-
   hale, and slowly re-
   turn to upright po-
   sition.
5. Repeat, leaning to the
   opposite side.

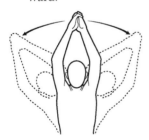

Arm Circles:
To relax the neck and up-
per back muscles

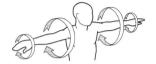

1. Stand or sit.
2. Raise your arms
   straight out to the side.
3. Slowly rotate your
   arms in small, then
   large circles.
4. Change directions.

IMPROVING MUSCLE STRENGTH AND DEXTERITY

Well-conditioned muscles have improved control and
endurance, allow for freer wrist movement, and reduce
the likelihood of injury. The hand is controlled by 35
muscles: 20 muscles in the hand itself and 15 muscles in
the forearm. These muscles are divided into four muscle
groups: (1) extensors that open the fingers, (2) flexor
muscles that close the fingers, (3) abductors that spread
the fingers, and (4) adductors that bring the fingers together. The most recommended form of exercise is one
that exercises all muscle pairs in the fingers and hand.

Hand Exercises

The hand exercises shown here use Power Putty, a silicone rubber material that resists squeezing and stretch-
ing forces. These hand exercises are reprinted with permission of *SportsHealth*. **Directions:** For each exercise
illustrated, squeeze or stretch the Power Putty for the
suggested number of repetitions. Begin with exercise
number one and proceed through to number nine without stopping. The exercise set, for both hands doing all
nine exercises, should take no more than 10 to 20
minutes. When exercising, maintain your hands at or
above waist level. Exercising with the hands hanging
down toward the feet will cause the blood to pool in
the vessels in the carpal tunnel of the wrist.

Caution: As with any exercise, don't do a hand exercise if it hurts. If you have or suspect that you may have a musculoskeletal injury, do not attempt these exercises without the permission of a physician.

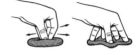

1. Full Grip (flexor muscles).

Squeeze putty with your fingers against the palm of your hand. Roll it over and around in your hand and repeat as rapidly and with as much strength as possible.

Suggested Repetitions: 10

2. All Finger Spread (extensor and abductor muscles).

Form putty into a thick pancake shape and place on a table top. Bunch fingertips together and place in putty. Spread fingers out as fast as possible.

Suggested Repetitions: 3

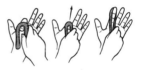

3. Fingers Dig (flexor muscles).

Place putty in the palm of your hand and dig fingertips deep into the putty. Release the fingers, roll putty over, and repeat.

Suggested Repetitions: 10

4. Finger Extension (extensor muscles).

Close one finger into palm of hand. Wrap putty over tip of finger and hold loose ends with the other hand. As quickly as possible, extend finger to a fully opened position. Regulate difficulty by increasing or decreasing thickness of putty wrapped over the fingertip. Repeat with each finger.

Suggested Repetitions: 3

5. Thumb Press (flexor muscles).
Form putty into a barrel shape and place in the palm of your hand. Press your thumb into the putty with as much force as you can. Reform putty and repeat.
Suggested Repetitions: 5

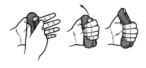

6. Thumb Extension (extensor muscles).
Bend your thumb toward the palm of the hand; wrap putty over the thumb tip. Hold the loose ends down and extend the thumb open as quickly as possible. Regulate difficulty by increasing or decreasing the thickness of putty wrapped over tip of thumb.
Suggested Repetitions: 3

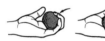

7. Fingers Only (flexor muscles).
Lay putty across fingers, and squeeze with fingertips only. Keep the palm of your hand flat and open. Rotate putty with thumb and repeat.
Suggested Repetitions: 10

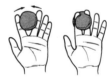

8. Finger Scissors (adductor muscles).
Form putty into the shape of a ball, and place between any two fingers. Squeeze fingers together in scissorslike motion. Repeat with each pair of fingers.
Suggested Repetitions: 3

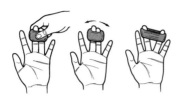

9. Finger Splits (abductor muscles).

Mold putty around any two fingers while they are closed together. Spread fingers apart as quickly as possible. Repeat exercise with each pair of fingers. Suggested Repetitions: 3

Power Putty is available in four levels of rigidity: soft, soft/medium, medium/firm, and hard. Power Putty can be purchased in sport stores or directly from: SportsHealth, 527 West Windsor Road, Glendale, California 91204 USA, (818) 240-7170.

Section 7:

References and Suggested Readings

Work-Related Musculoskeletal Disorders

Akesson, I., Lundborg, G., Horstmann, V., Skerfving, S.: Neuropathy in female dental personnel exposed to high frequency vibrations. Occup Environ Med Feb;52(2):116-23, 1995.

American Health Consultants. How to avoid carpal tunnel syndrome in daily practice. GP 2:134-140, 1993.

Atwood, M.J., Michalak, C.: The occurrence of cumulative trauma in dental hygienists. Work: A Journal of Prevention, Assessment, and Rehabilitation 2, 17, Summer, 1992.

Barry, R.M., Woodall, W.R., Mahan, J.M.: Postural changes in dental hygienists, four year longitudinal study. J Dent Hyg Mar-Apr;66:147-50, 1992.

Boyer, E.M., Elton, J., Preston, K.: Precautionary procedures—use in dental hygiene practice. Dent Hyg 60:516, 1986.

Brogmus, G.E., Sorock, G.S., Webster, B.S.: Recent trends in work-related cumulative trauma disorders of the upper extremities in the United States: An evaluation of possible reasons. J Occup Environ Med Apr;38(4):401-11, 1996.

Byl, N.N., Melnick, M: The neural consequences of repetition: clinical implications of a learning hypothesis. J Hand Ther Apr-Jun;10(2):160-74, 1997.

Centers for Disease Control: Occupational disease surveillance: Carpal tunnel syndrome. JAMA 262:886, 1989.

Centers for Disease Control: Occupational disease surveillance: carpal tunnel syndrome. MMWR Morb Mortal Wkly Rep 38:485-9, 1989.

Colangelo, G.A., Hobart, D.J., Belenky, M.M., Bechtel, R.H.: Elbow angle during a simulated task requiring fine psychomotor control. J Dent Educ Dec;55(12):785-8, 1991.

Conrad, J.C., Conrad, K.J., Osborn, J.B.: A short-term, three-year epidemiological study of median nerve sensitivity in practicing dental hygienists. J Dent Hyg Jul-Aug;67(5):268-72, 1993.

Conrad, J.C., Conrad, K.J., Osborn, J.: Median nerve dysfunction evaluated during dental hygiene education and practice (1986-1989). J Dent Hyg Jul-Aug;65(6):283-8, 1991.

Conrad, J.C., Conrad, K.J., Osborn, J.: Median nerve dysfunction evaluated during dental hygiene education and practice (1986-1989). J Dent Hyg Jul-Aug;65(6):283-8, 1991.

Cooper, M.D., Brian, J.N.: Musculoskeletal exercises for the dental professional. Dent Hyg News 8(4), 17-8, 1996.

DeStefano, F., Nordstrom, D.L., Vierkant, R.A.: Long-term symptom outcomes of carpal tunnel syndrome and its treatment. J Hand Surg Am Mar;22(2):200-10, 1997.

Douglas, D.D.: OSHA's proposed ergonomic standard: is it necessary for dentistry? AGD Impact 20-1, 1994.

Ekberg, K., Karlsson, M., Axelson, O., Malm, P.: Cross-sectional study of
    risk factors for symptoms in the neck and shoulder area. Ergonomics
    May;38(5):971-80, 1995.
Ekberg, K., Bjorkqvist, B., Malm, P., Bjerre-Kiely, B., Karlsson, M., Axelson,
    O.: Case-control study of risk factors for disease in the neck and
    shoulder area. Occup Environ Med Apr;51(4):262-6, 1994.
Fernstrom E.A., Ericson, M.O.: Upper-arm elevation during office work.
    Ergonomics Oct;39(10):1221-30, 1996.
Frederick, L.J., Armstrong, T.J.: Effect of friction and load on pinch force in a
    hand transfer task. Ergonomics Dec;38(12):2447-54, 1995.
Garfunkel, A.A., Galili, D.: Dental health care workers at risk. Dent Clin
    North Am Apr;40(2):277-91, 1996.
Gorton, C.: An ounce of prevention. . . . RDH Sep;14(9):26-8, 1994.
Haag, A.B.: Ergonomic standards, guidelines, and strategies for prevention
    of back injury. Occup Med Jan-Mar;7(1):155-65, 1992.
Hamlin, C., Hitchcock, M., Hofmeister, J., Owens, R.: Predicting surgical
    outcome for pain relief and return to work. [corrected and repub-
    lished article originally printed in Best Pract Benchmarking Health
    1996 Sep-Oct;1(5):258-61]. Best Pract Benchmarking Health Nov-
    Dec;1(6):311-4, 1996.
Hudson, A.R., Wissinger, J.P., Salazar, J.L., Kline, D.G., Yarzagaray, L.,
    Danoff, D., Fernandez, E., Field, E.M., Gainsburg, D.B., Fabi, R.A.,
    Mackinnon, S.E.: Carpal tunnel syndrome. Surg Neurol
    Feb;47(2):105-14, 1997.
Hunt, C.M.: How to manage cumulative trauma injuries in dental labora-
    tories. Trends Tech Contemp Dent Lab Jul-Aug;11(6):23-6, 1994.
Jacobsen, N., Derand, T., Hensten-Pettersen, A.: Profile of work-related
    health complaints among Swedish dental laboratory technicians.
    Community Dent Oral Epidemiol Apr;24(2):138-44, 1996.
Jacobsen, N., Hensten-Pettersen, A.: Occupational health problems among
    dental hygienists. Community Dent Oral Epidemiol Jun;23(3):177-
    81, 1995.
Keyserling, W.M., Stetson, D.S., Silverstein, B.A., Brouwer, M.L.: A check-
    list for evaluating ergonomic risk factors associated with upper ex-
    tremity cumulative trauma disorders. Ergonomics Jul;36(7):807-31,
    1993.
King, P.M.: Sensory function assessment. A pilot comparison study of touch
    pressure threshold with texture and tactile discrimination. J Hand Ther
    Jan-Mar;10(1):24-8, 1997.
Latko, W.A., Armstrong, T.J., Foulke, J.A., Herrin, G.D., Rabourn, RA., Ulin,
    S.S.: Development and evaluation of an observational method for as-
    sessing repetition in hand tasks. Am Ind Hyg Assoc J Apr;58(4):278-
    85, 1997.
Liskiewicz, S.T., Kerschbaum, W.E.: Cumulative trauma disorders: An ergo-
    nomic approach for prevention. J Dent Hyg Summer;71(4):162-7,
    1997.
Lundstrom, R., Nilsson, T., Burstrom, L., Hagberg, M.: Vibrotactile percep-
    tion sensitivity and its relation to hand-arm vibration exposure. Cent
    Eur J Public Health 3 Suppl:62-5, 1995.
Marley, R., et al.: Thompson dental tool study final report. University Techni-
    cal Assistance Program, April 10, 1995.

Mercer, R.B., Marcella, C.P., Carney, D.K., McDonaldm R.W.: Occupational health hazards to the ultrasonographer and their possible prevention. J Am Soc Echocardiogr May;10(4):363-6, 1997.

Moen, B.E., Bjorvatn, K.: Musculoskeletal symptoms among dentists in a dental school. Occup Med Oxf Feb;46(1):65-8, 1996.

Morganstein, W.: Performance logic, the ultimate application. J Dent Prac Admin 2:31, 1984.

Nakladalova, M., Fialova, J., Korycanova, H., Nakladal, Z.: State of health in dental technicians with regard to vibration exposure and overload of upper extremities. Cent Eur J Public Health 3 Suppl:129-31, 1995.

Novak, C.B., Mackinnon, S.E.: Repetitive use and static postures: a source of nerve compression and pain. J Hand Ther Apr-Jun;10(2):151-9, 1997.

Nunn, P.F.: Getting a handle on ergonomic periodontal instrument design. Access, Americam Dental Hygienists' Association Mar;11(3):16-9, 1997.

Nunn, P., Hart, C., Gaulden, F.: 'Perfect' instrumentation can be hazardous to your health or ergonomic applications for the prevention of carpal tunnel syndrome. Access, American Dental Hygienists' Association, 9: 37-43, January 1995.

Öberg, T., Karsznia, A., Sandsjo, L., Kadefors, R.: Work load, fatigue, and pause patterns in clinical dental hygiene. J Dent Hyg Sep-Oct;69(5):223-9, 1995.

Öberg, T.: Ergonomic evaluation and construction of a reference workplace in dental hygiene: A case study. J Dent Hyg July-Aug;67(5):262-67, 1993.

Occhipinti, E., Colombini, D., Molteni, G., Grieco, A.: Criteria for the ergonomic evaluation of work chairs. Med Lav Jul-Aug;84(4):274-85, 1993.

Pecina, M.M., Krmpotic-Nemanic, J., Markiewitz, A.D.: Tunnel syndromes: Peripheral nerve compression syndromes, 2nd ed. Boca Raton: CRC Press Inc., 1996.

Poindexter, S. M.: All the right moves: Ergonomics & the dental hygienist at work. Access, American Dental Hygienists' Association, Jan;9;18-33, 1995.

Pollack, R.: Dento-ergonomics: the key to energy-saving performance. J Calif Dent Assoc Apr;24(4):63-6, 68, 1996.

Pollack, R.: Dental office ergonomics: how to reduce stress factors and increase efficiency. J Can Dent Assoc Jun;62(6):508-10, 1996.

Powell B.J., Winkley, G.P., Brown, J.O., Etersque, S.: Evaluating the fit of ambidextrous and fitted gloves: implications for hand discomfort. J Am Dent Assoc Sep;125:1235-42, 1994.

Radecki, P.: A gender specific wrist ratio and the likelihood of median nerve abnormality at the carpal tunnel. Am J Phys Med Rehabil 73(3), 1994.

Ranney, D.: Work-related chronic injuries of the forearm and hand: Their specific diagnosis and management. Ergonomics 36(8):871-80, 1993.

Rayan, G.M.: Proximal ulnar nerve compression. Hand Clin 8(2):325-36, 1992.

Rempel, D., Keir, P.J., Smutz, W.P., Hargens, A.: Effects of static fingertip
    loading on carpal tunnel pressure. J Orthop Res May;15(3):422-6,
    1997.
Rempel, D., Manojlovic, R., Levinsohn, D.G., Bloom, T., Gordon, L.: The ef-
    fect of wearing a flexible wrist splint on carpal tunnel pressure during
    repetitive hand activity. J Hand Surg 19A:106-09, 1994.
Rhode, J.: Ambidextrous gloves—can they contribute to carpal tunnel syn-
    drome? Dentistry Today 9:1-2, 1990.
Robinson, M.: Home position dentistry: the beach philosophy of dental prac-
    tice. Kyoto, Japan, Bikensha Co., 1976.
Rohmert, W., Wos, H., Norlander, S., Helbig, R.: Effects of vibration on
    arm and shoulder muscles in three body postures. Eur J Appl Physiol
    59:243-8, 1989.
Rundcrantz, B.L., Johnsson, B., Moritz, U.: Pain and discomfort in the muscu-
    loskeletal system among dentists. A prospective study. Swed Dent J
    15(5):219-28, 1991.
Rundcrantz, B.L., Johnsson, B., Moritz, U.: Occupational cervico-brachial
    disorders among dentists. Analysis of ergonomics and locomotor
    functions. Swed Dent J 15(3):105-15, 1991.
Scheer, S.J., Mital, A.: Ergonomics. Arch Phys Med Rehabil Mar;78(3
    Suppl):S36-45, 1997.
Shevach, A., Berg, R.G., Berkley, D.B., Mann, J.: Ergonomics and health
    considerations at chairside. Dental Teamwork Nov-Dec;9(6), 10-4,
    1996.
Silverstein, B.A., Stetson, D.S., Keyserling, W.M., Fine, L.J.: Work-related
    musculoskeletal disorders: comparison of data sources for surveil-
    lance. Am J Ind Med May;31(5):600-8, 1997.
Snook, S.H., Vaillancourt, D.R., Ciriello, V.M., Webster, B.S.: Maximum
    acceptable forces for repetitive ulnar deviation of the wrist. Am Ind
    Hyg Assoc J Jul;58(7):509-17, 1997.
Snook, S.H., Vaillancourt, D.R., Ciriello, V.M., Webster, B.S.: Psychophysi-
    cal studies of repetitive wrist flexion and extension. Ergonomics
    Jul;38(7):1488-507, 1995.
SportsHealth: Hand exercises with therapy putty. Glendale, CA: Sports-
    Health.
Sprouls, L.S.: Carpal tunnel syndrome. Preventing a malady of repeated mo-
    tion. Dent Teamwork Jul-Aug 1993.
Stallings, S.P., Kasdan, M.L., Soergel, T.M., Corwin, H.M.: A case-control
    study of obesity as a risk factor for carpal tunnel syndrome in a popu-
    lation of 600 patients presenting for independent medical examina-
    tion. J Hand Surg Am Mar;22(2):211-5, 1997.
Stenz, T.L., Riley, M.W., Harn, S.D., Sposate, R.C., Stockstill, J.W., Harn,
    J.A.: Upper extremity altered sensations in dental hygienists. Industrial
    Ergonomics Apr;13(2), 107, 1994.
Tatro, D.E.: Ergonomics for the dental hygienist. Practical Hygiene Jan-
    Feb;6(1), 35-9, 1997.
Thomas, R.E., Vaidya, S.C., Herrick, R.T., Congleton, J.J.: The effects of bio-
    feedback on carpal tunnel syndrome. Ergonomics Apr;36(4):353-
    61, 1993.
Thomas, R.E., Butterfield, R.K, Hool, J.N., Herrick, R.T.: Effects of exercise
    on carpal tunnel symptoms. Applied Ergonomics 24(2), 101-8,
    1993.

UAW-GM Human Resource Center: Ergonomics handbook. UAW-GM Human Resource Center, April 1988.

U.S. Department of Health and Human Services, Public Health Service, Centers for Disease Control, National Institute for Occupational Safety and Health. Carpal tunnel syndrome: Selected references, 1989.

U.S. Dept. of Health and Human Services. The international classification of diseases—(9th revision) clinical modification—ICD-9-CM DHHS, (PHS)#89-1260, 3(1):275-772, 1989.

Vessey, M.P., Villard-Mackintosh, L., Yeates, D.: Epidemiology of carpal tunnel syndrome in women of childbearing age. Findings in a large cohort study. Int J Epidemiol 19(3):655-9, 1990.

Visser J.L., Straker, L.M.: An investigation of discomfort experienced by dental therapists and assistants at work. Aust Dent J Feb;39(1):39-44, 1994.

Werner, R.A., Franzblau, A., Albers, J.W., Buchele, H., Armstrong, T.J.: Use of screening nerve conduction studies for predicting future carpal tunnel syndrome. Occup Environ Med Feb;54(2):96-100, 1997.

Werner, R.A., Franzblau, A.: Hand dominance effect on median and ulnar sensory evoked amplitude and latency in asymptomatic workers. Arch Phys Med Rehabil May;77(5):473-6, 1996.

White, D.J., Cox, E.R., Bacca, L., Lanzalaco, A.C., Montgomery, R.M., Coyle-Rees, M., Beiswanger, B.B., Mau, M., Arends, J.: A Quanticalc clinical comparison of professional efficiency in manual supragingival calculus debridement. J Clin Dent 7(2 Spec No):54-7, 1996.

White, D.J., Cox, E.R., Arends, J., Nieborg, J.H., Leydsman, H., Wieringa, D.W., Dijkman, A.G., Ruben, J.R.: Instruments and methods for the quantitative measurement of factors affecting hygienist/dentist efforts during scaling and root planing of the teeth. J Clin Dent 7(2 Spec No):32-40, 1996.

Wolfe, F.: The sensible thing to do is prevent the pain. RDH May;17(5), 34, 36, 54, 1997.

Yassi, A.: Repetitive strain injuries. Lancet Mar 29;349(9056):943-7, 1997.

Young, J.M.: Ergonomic considerations in the dental laboratory environment. Trends Tech Contemp Dent Lab Jul-Aug;11(6):17-20, 1994.

Zabel, A.M., McGrew, A.B.: Ergonomics. A key component in a CTD control program. AAOHN J Jul;45(7):350-8; quiz 359-60, 1997.

Glove Use and Latex Sensitivity:

Academy of General Dentistry. Dental workers and latex allergy. OSHAlert Winter 3(1): 1-7, 1997.

Albin, M.S., Bunegin, L., Duke, E.S., Ritter, R.R., Page, C.P.: Anatomy of a defective barrier: sequential glove leak detection in a surgical and dental environment. Crit Care Med Feb;20(2):170-84, 1992.

American Association of Nurse Anesthetists. Latex allergy protocol. J Am Assoc Nurse Anesthetists 61;223-4, 1993.

Baggett, F.J., Burke, F.J., Wilson, N.H.: An assessment of the incidence of punctures in gloves when worn for routine operative procedures. Br Dent J Jun 5;174(11):412-6, 1993.

Baumann, M.A.: The influence of dental gloves on the setting of impression materials. Br Dent J Aug 19;179(4):130-5, 1995.

Beezhold, D.H., Sussman, G.L., Liss, G.M., Chang, N.S.: Latex allergy can induce clinical reactions to specific foods. Clin Exp Allergy Apr;26(4):416-22, 1995.

Beezhold, D.H., Kostyal, D.A., Wiseman, J.: The transfer of protein allergens from latex gloves: a study of influencing factors. AORN J 59:605-13, 1994.

Bensky, K.P.: Latex allergy: who, what, when, where, why, and how. CRNA Nov;6(4):177-82, 1995.

Berg, G.A., Kirk, A.J., Bain, W.H.: Punctured surgical gloves and bacterial re-colonisation of hands during open heart surgery: implications for prosthetic valve replacement. Br J Clin Pract Sep;41(9):903-6, 1987.

Bernstein, M.: An overview of latex allergy and its implications for emergency nurses. J Emerg Nurs 22:29-36, 1996.

Booth, B.: Latex allergy: a growing problem in health care. Prof Nurse Feb;11(5):316, 318-9, 1996.

Boyer, E.M.: The effectiveness of a low-chemical, low-protein medical glove to prevent or reduce dermatological problems. J Dent Hyg Mar-Apr;69(2):67-73, 1995.

Brugnami, G., Brugnami G., Marabini, A., Siracusa, A., Abbritti, G.: Work-related late asthmatic response induced by latex allergy. J Allergy Clin Immunol Oct;96(4):457-64, 1995.

Burke, F.J., Wilson N.H.: Orofacial reactions after contact with latex gloves. Br Dent J Nov 23;181(10):361, 1996.

Burke, F.J., Wilson, M.A., McCord, J.F.: Allergy to latex gloves in clinical practice: case reports. Quintessence Int Dec;26(12):859-63, 1995.

Centers for Disease Control: Recommendations for prevention of HIV transmission in health-care settings. MMWR Morb Mortal Wkly Rep 36 (Suppl 2S): 2S-18S, 1987.

Charous, B.L., Banov, C., Yassin, M. (Latex Hypersensitivity Committee): Latex allergy—an emerging healthcare problem. Ann Allergy Asthma Immunol July;75(1):19-21, 1995.

Charous, B.L., Hamilton, R.G., Yunginger, J.W.: Occupational latex exposure: characteristics of contact and systemic reactions in 47 workers. J Allergy Clin Immunol Jul;94(1):12-8, 1994.

Chen, H.D., Chen, C.L., Huang, S.W.: Characterization of latex allergens and correlation of serum IgE/IgG antibody ratio with clinical symptoms. Allergy Asthma Proc May-Jun;17(3):143-8, 1996.

Conde-Salazar, L., del-Rio, E., Guimaraens, D., et al.: Type IV allergy to rubber additives: A 10-year study of 686 cases. J Am Acad Derm 29:176-80, 1993.

Cormio, L., Turjanmaa, K., Talja, M., Andersson, L.C., Ruutu, M.: Toxicity and immediate allergenicity of latex gloves. Clin Exp Allergy 23:618-23, 1993.

Cotter, C.M., Burbach, C., Boyer, M., Engelhardt, M., Smith, M., Hubka, K.: Latex allergy and the student with spina bifida. J Sch Nurs Oct;12(3):14-8, 1996.

Delbourg, M.F., Guilloux, L., Moneret-Vautrin, D.A., Ville, G.: Hypersensitivity to banana in latex-allergic patients. Identification of two major banana allergens of 33 and 37 kD. Ann Allergy Asthma Immunol Apr;76(4):321-6, 1996.

Delbourg, M.F., Guilloux, L., Moneret-Vautrin, D.A., Ville, G.: Hypersensitivity to latex and Ficus benjamina allergens. Ann Allergy Asthma Immunol Dec;75(6 Pt1):496-500, 1995.

Dillard, S.F., MacCollurn M.A.: Reports to FDA: Allergic reactions to latex containing medical devices. International latex conference: Sensitivity to latex in medical devices. Nov, 1992.

Emans, J.B.: Allergy to latex in patients who have myelodysplasia. Relevance for the orthopaedic surgeon. J Bone Joint Surg Am Aug;74(7):1103-9, 1992.

Escoe, R.: Electrical permeability of latex gloves. N Y State Dent J Jan;61(1):37-9, 1995.

Fein, J.A., Fein JA., Selbst, S.M., Pawlowski, N.A.: Latex allergy in pediatric emergency department personnel. Pediatr Emerg Care Feb;12(1):6-9, 1996.

Field, E.A.: The use of powdered gloves in dental practice: a cause for concern? J Dent May-Jul;25(3-4):209-14, 1997.

Field, E.A.: Hypoallergenic gloves. Int Dent J Dec;45(6):339-46, 1995.

Field, E.A.: Implications of hand dermatitis for dental education. J Dent Educ Aug;59(8):821-3, 1995.

Field, E.A., Fay, M.F.: Issues of latex safety in dentistry. Br Dent J Oct 7;179(7):247-53, 1995.

Food and Drug Administration: Allergic reactions to latex-containing medical devices, March 29, 1991 (MDA 91-1). Rockville, MD: U.S. Department of Health and Human Services, 1991.

Freeman, G.L.: Concurrence of latex and fruit allergies. Allergy Asthma Proc Mar-Apr;18(2):85-8, 1997.

Friesen, C.D., O'Connell, M., Schkade, P.A., Dyer, P.D.: Latex-induced asthma in a dental assistant. Gen Dent Sep-Oct;44(5):424-6, 1996.

Grandy, L., Slater, J.: The history and diagnosis of latex allergy. Immunol Allergy Clin North Am: Latex Allergy Feb;15(1), 1995.

Grzybowski, M., Ownby, D.R., Peyser, P.A., Johnson, C.C., Schork, M.A.: The prevalence of anti-latex IgE antibodies among registered nurses. J Allergy Clin Immunol Sep;98(3):535-44, 1996.

Hamann, B., Hamann, C., Taylor, J.S.: Managing latex allergies in the dental office. J Calif Dent Assoc Jan;23(1):45-50, 1995.

Hamann, C.P., Kick, S.A.: Allergies associated with medical gloves. Manufacturing issues. Dermatol Clin Jul;12(3):547-59, 1994.

Huang, S.W.: Latex allergy: a new threat to patients and health professionals. J Formos Med Assoc May;95(5):361-3, 1996.

Hunt, L.W., Fransway, A.F., Reed, C.E., Miller, L.K., Jones, R.T., Swanson, M.C., Yunginger, J.W.: An epidemic of occupational allergy to latex involving health care workers. J Occup Environ Med Oct;37(10):1204-9, 1995.

Hunt, L.W., Boone-Orke, J.L., Fransway, A.F., Fremstad, C.E., Jones, R.T., Swanson, M.C., McEvoy, M.T., Miller, L.K., Majerus, E.T., Luker, PA., Scheppmann, D.L., Webb, M.J., Yunginger, J.W.: A medical-center-wide, multidisciplinary approach to the problem of natural rubber latex allergy. J Occup Environ Med Aug;38(8):765-770, 1996.

Jackson, D.: Latex allergy and anaphylaxis—what to do? J Intraven Nurs Jan-Feb;18(1):33-52, 1995.

Jezierski, M.: ELASTIC and ALERT: help for nurses and others with latex allergies, help for those who work with latex. Education for latex allergy/support team and information coalition. Allergy to Latex Education and Resource Team. J Emerg Nurs Apr;23(2):43A-45A, 1997.

Jones, J.M., Sussman, G.L., Beezhold, D.H.: Latex allergen levels of injectable collagen stored in syringes with rubber plungers. Urology Jun;47(6):898-902, 1996.

Kam, P.C., Thompson, J.F.: Latex allergy: an emerging health hazard for operating theatre staff. Br J Surg Mar;84(3):289-90, 1997.

Katelaris, C.H., Widmer, R.P., Lazarus, R.M.: Prevalence of latex allergy in a dental school. Med J Aust Jun 17;164(12):711-4, 1996.

Kellett, P.B.: Latex allergy: a review. J Emerg Nurs Feb;23(1):27-34; quiz 34-6, 1997.

Kelly, K.: Management of the latex-allergic patient. Immunol Allergy Clin North Am: Latex Allergy 15(1), Feb 1995.

Kelly, K.: Stop the sensitization. Source Surg Newslett Feb;3(1), 1995.

Kelly, K.J.: Diagnosis of latex allergy. Source Surg 3:4, 1995.

Kinnaird, S.W., Kinnaird SW., McClure, N., Wilham, S.: Latex allergy: an emerging problem in health care. Neonatal Netw Oct;14(7):33-8, 1995.

Korniewicz, D.: Barrier protection of latex. Immunol Allergy Clin North Am: Latex Allergy Feb;15(1), 1995.

Korniewicz, D.M., Kelly, K.J.: Barrier protection and latex allergy associated with surgical gloves. AORN J Jun;61(6):1037-40, 1043-4, 1995.

Korniewicz, D.M., Garzon, L.S.: How to choose and use gloves. Nursing Sep;24(9):18, 1994.

Kotilainen, H.R., Avato, J.L., Gantz, N.M.: Latex and vinyl nonsterile examination gloves: status report on laboratory evaluation of defects by physical and biological methods. Appl Environ Microbiol Jun;56(6):1627-30, 1990.

Lagier, F., Vervloet, D., Lhermet, I., Poyen, D., Charpin, D.: Prevalence of latex allergy in operating room nurses. J Allergy Clin Immunol 90:319-22, 1992.

Landwehr, L.P., Boguniewicz, M.: Current perspectives of latex allergy. J Pediatrics Mar;128(3):305-12, 1996.

Lavaud, F., Prevost, A., Cossart, C., Guerin, L., Bernard J., Kochman, S.: Allergy to latex, avocado pear, and banana: evidence for a 30 kd antigen in immunoblotting. J Allergy Clin Immunol Feb;95(2):557-64, 1995.

Leger, R., Meeropol, E.: Children at risk: latex allergy and spina bifida. J Pediatric Nurs 21:38-9, 1992.

Liebke, C., Niggemann, B., Wahn, U.: Sensitivity and allergy to latex in atopic and non-atopic children. Pediatr Allergy Immunol May;7(2):103-7, 1996.

Liss, G.M., Sussman, G.L., Deal, K., Brown, S., Cividino, M., Siu, S., Beezhold, D.H., Smith, G., Swanson, M.C., Yunginger, J., Douglas, A.,Holness, D.L., Lebert, P., Keith, P., Wasserman, S., Turjanmaa,

K.: Latex allergy: epidemiological study of 1351 hospital workers. Occup Environ Med May;54(5):335-42, 1997.

Lu, L.J., Kurup, V.P., Hoffman, D.R., Kelly, K.J., Murali, P.S., Fink, J.N.: Characterization of a major latex allergen associated with hypersensitivity in spina bifida patients. J Immunol Sep 1;155(5):2721-8, 1995.

Lu, L.J., Kurup, V.P., Fink, J.N., Kelly, K.J.: Comparison of latex antigens from surgical gloves, ammoniated and nonammoniated latex: effect of ammonia treatment on natural rubber latex proteins. J Lab Clin Med Aug;126(2):161-8, 1995.

Mansell, P., Reckless, J.P., Lovell, C.R.: Severe anaphylactic reaction to latex rubber surgical gloves. Br Dent J Feb 11;178(3):86-7, 1995.

McCormack, B., Cameron, M., Biel, L: Latex sensitivity: an occupational health strategic plan. AAOHN J Apr;43(4):190-6, 1995.

Melton, A.L.: Managing latex allergy in patients and health care workers. Cleve Clin J Med Feb;64(2):76-82, 1997.

Merchant, V.A., Molinari, J.A., Pickett, T.: Microbial penetration of gloves following usage in routine dental procedures. Am J Dent Apr;5(2):95-6, 1992.

Michael, T., Niggemann, B., Moers, A., Seidel, U., Wahn, U., Scheffner, D.: Risk factors for latex allergy in patients with spina bifida. Clin Exp Allergy Aug;26(8):934-9, 1996.

Molinari, J.A.: Emerging infection-control issues: increasing incidence of latex hypersensitivity. Compend Contin Educ Dent Apr;16(4):346, 348, 1995.

Moore, M.: Poor production methods may encourage reactions. Rubber and Plastics News November 23;4, 1992.

Munksgaard, E.C., Hansen, E.K., Engen, T., Holm, U.: Self-reported occupational dermatological reactions among Danish dentists. Eur J Oral Sci Aug;104(4):396-402, 1996.

Nelson, L.P., Soporowski, N.J., Shusterman, S.: Latex allergies in children with spina bifida: relevance for the pediatric dentist. Pediatr Dent Jan-Feb;16(1):18-22, 1994.

O'Neale, M.: Petrolatum ointment and gloving. AORN J 52(3):612, 1990.

Ozata, F., Sepetcioglu, F., Turkun, M., Eltem, R.: Permeability of protective gloves used in dental practice. Quintessence Int Mar;25(3):181-4, 1994.

Porri, F., Lemiere, C., Birnbaum, J., Guilloux, L., Lanteaume, A., Didelot, R., Vervloet, D., Charpin, D.: Prevalence of latex sensitization in subjects attending health screening: implications for a perioperative screening. Clin Exp Allergy Apr;27(4):413-7, 1997.

Porri, F., Pradal, M., Lemiere, C., Birnbaum, J., Mege, J.L., Lanteaume, A., Charpin, D., Vervloet, D., Camboulives, J.: Association between latex sensitization and repeated latex exposure in children. Anesthesiology Mar;86(3):599-602, 1997.

Rankin, K.V, Seale, N.S., Jones, D.L., Rees, T.D.: Reported latex sensitivity in pediatric dental patients from hospital- and dental school-based populations. Pediatr Dent Mar-Apr;16(2):117-20, 1994.

Ready, M.A., Schuster, G.S., Wilson, J.T., Hanes, C.M.: Effects of dental medicaments on examination glove permeability. J Prosth Dent 61:4, 1989.

Richards, J.M., Sydiskis, R.J., Davidson, W.M., Stuart, D.J., Lavine, D.S.: Permeability of latex gloves after contact with dental materials. Am J Orthod 104:224-9, 1993.

Roy, A., Epstein, J., Onno, E.: Latex allergies in dentistry: recognition and recommendations. J Can Dent Assoc Apr;63(4):297-300, 1997.

Safadi, G.S., Safadi, T.J., Terezhalmy, G.T., Taylor, J.S., Battisto, J.R., Melton, A.L.: Latex hypersensitivity: its prevalence among dental professionals. J Am Dent Assoc Jan;127(1):83-8, 1996.

Safadi, G.S., Safadi, T.J., Terezhalmy, G., Melton, A.L.: Latex hypersensitivity: a study of prevalence in a dental practice. American College of Allergy & Immunology, 1994.

Shah, M., Lewis, F.M., Gawkrodger, D.J.: Delayed and immediate orofacial reactions following contact with rubber gloves during dental treatment. Br Dent J Aug 24;181(4):137-9, 1996.

Sorva, R., Makinen-Kiljunen, S., Suvilehto, K., Juntunen-Backman, K., Haahtela, T.: Latex allergy in children with no known risk factor for latex sensitization. Pediatr Allergy Immunol Feb;6(1):36-8, 1995.

Strzyzewski, N.M.: Latex allergy: everyone is at risk. Plast Surg Nurs Winter;15(4):204-6, 1995.

Sussman, G.L., Gold, M.: Guidelines for the Management of Latex Allergies and safe latex use in health care facilities. American College of Allergy, Asthma & Immunology March 1966.

Tarlo, S.M., Sussman, G.L., Holness, D.L.: Latex sensitivity in dental students and staff: a cross-sectional study. J Allergy Clin Immunol Mar;99(3):396-401, 1997.

Tinsley, D., Chadwick, R.G.: The permeability of dental gloves following exposure to certain dental materials. J Dent Jan;25(1):65-70, 1997.

Truscott, W.: They're not just gloves: a guideline on proper use. CDS Rev Mar;88(2):22-9, 1995.

Truscott, W.: Reactions to natural rubber latex. First Hand, Safeskin Corporation, Educational Series 1, 1, 1994.

Truscott, W.: Issues with regards to post-cure processing. Safeskin Corporation, Educational Series 1994.

Truscott, W.: Glove powder: Friend or foe? First Hand, Safeskin Corporation, Educational Series 1, 2, 1994.

Vassallo, S.A., Kim, S.H., Todres, I.D.: Latex allergy and plastic syringes. Anesth Analg Feb;428-9, 1996.

Vassallo, S.A., Thurston, T.A., Kim, S.H, Todres, I.D.: Allergic reaction to latex from stopper of a medication vial. Anesth Analg 80:1057-8, 1995.

Vogel, L.C., Schrader, T., Lubicky, J.P.: Latex allergy in children and adolescents with spinal cord injuries. J Pediatr Orthop Jul-Aug;15(4):517-20, 1995.

Williams, P.B., Buhr, M.P., Weber, R.W., Volz, M.A., Koepke, J.W., Selner, J.C.: Latex allergen in respirable particulate air pollution. J Allergy Clin Immunol 95:88-93, 1995.

2

Periodontal Assessment

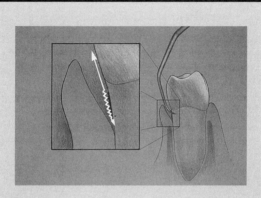

In this chapter

Section 3:

Assessments with Explorers

- Types of Explorers
- Technique for Use of a Universal Explorer
- Interpretation of Subgingival Conditions
- Mechanic's Check: Common Causes of Undetected Calculus
- Use of an Explorer for Caries Detection
- Technique for Caries Detection

Section 4:

Periodontal Screening and Recording System

Section 5:

Communicating Findings to Patients—Intraoral Imaging Systems

Section 6:

References and Suggested Readings

Section 1:

Introduction to Periodontal Assessment Techniques

Successful nonsurgical therapy depends on a comprehensive assessment of the patient: (1) before treatment, (2) during and after instrumentation, and (3) following the initial therapy. A comprehensive patient assessment involves gathering the personal, comprehensive health, and medical histories of the patient and assessing all aspects of the periodontium and teeth.

An assessment of periodontal health status should include the following components.

1. **Cursory Examination**
A periodontal assessment should begin with a cursory examination of the mouth. Examine the patient's mouth for lesions, ulcerations, or areas of tissue trauma that may require consultation or would preclude further treatment at this time.

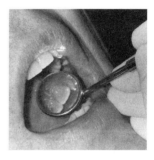

2. **Description of Gingival Tissues; Visual Signs of Inflammation**
Evaluate the color, shape, size, and contour of the gingival tissues.

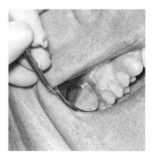

3. Tissue texture and consistency

Assess the texture and consistency of the free and attached tissues.

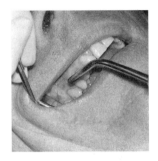

4. Tissue texture and consistency

Compressed air directed into the gingival sulcus or pocket is helpful in determining tissue consistency. In healthy individuals, the free gingiva is elastic and will remain adapted to the tooth.

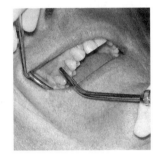

In patients with acute disease conditions, the tissue is flaccid and easily deflected away from the tooth by the stream of air. In patients with chronic disease, the tissue may be fibrotic and will not be displaced by the air.

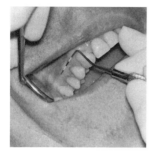

5. Tissue texture and consistency

The consistency of the attached gingiva is evaluated with a periodontal probe. Place a periodontal probe lengthwise across the attached gingiva, and apply gentle pressure against the tissue. Lift the probe away and observe the tissue response. The slight indentation and blanching of tissue color will quickly disappear if the tissue is healthy.

If the tissue is edematous, the blanching and indentation will remain evident for seconds. The probe will not produce an indentation in fibrotic tissue, and there will be little or no blanching of the tissue color.

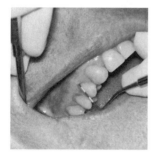

6. Clinical Attachment Level, Bleeding Points, Presence of Exudate, and the Position of the Gingival Margin

The probe is used around the circumference of each sulcus or pocket to assess the attachment level. The presence of bleeding or exudate should also be recorded.

The position of the gingival margin may be indicated by a line drawn on the anatomic chart or it may be recorded in numerical form as the distance in millimeters from the cementoenamel junction (CEJ).

7. Furcation Involvement

If indicated, a furcation probe is used to detect and classify furcation involvement.

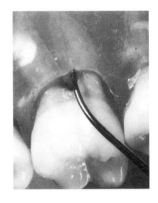

8. Mucogingival Examination

Subtract the probing depth from the total width of the gingiva to determine the width of the attached gingiva.

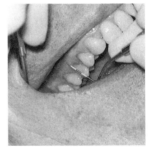

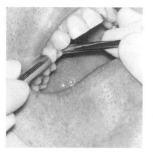

9. Examine the Teeth for Mobility

Each tooth in the sextant should be evaluated for the presence of mobility. All teeth have slight normal mobility because of the periodontal ligament. Mobility is assessed by applying alternating pressure with instrument handles, first from the facial aspect, then from the lingual aspect of the tooth.

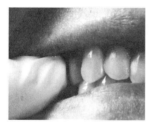

10. Check for Fremitus

Fremitus is tooth movement created by the patient's occlusal force while biting. The assessment is performed by placing your fingertip on the facial surface of the maxillary tooth as the patient taps the teeth together. Feel for vibration (i.e., movement) of the tooth.

COMMON CLINICAL VARIATIONS IN GINGIVAL TONE

Healthy Tissue	• No inflammation • Firm tissue tone • Tone is elastic: tissue springs back almost immediately if pressure is applied to it • No bleeding, no exudate
Edematous Tissue	• Acute inflammation • Spongy and engorged tissue tone • Red, purplish tissue color • Tone is nonelastic; if pressure is applied to tissue with side of probe the tissue will retain imprint of probe for several seconds • Spontaneous bleeding evident at margin on gentle probing • Exudate not typically present
Fibrotic Tissue	• Chronic inflammation • Rigid, dense tissue tone • Pale pink tissue color • Excessive stippling • Tone is nonelastic; the tissue is hard and resists imprint of probe if pressure is applied to tissue with side of probe • Exudate may be present

Common Clinical Variations in **Marginal Contour**

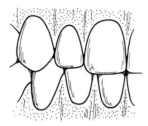

Normal contour: knife-edged, closely adapted to tooth surface

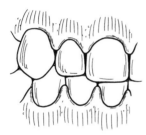

Abnormal contour: enlarged, rolled margins

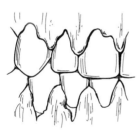

Abnormal contour: enlarged, irregular margins

Abnormal contour: margins festooned

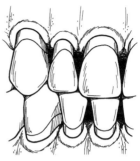

Abnormal contour: cleft margins

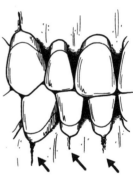

Common Clinical Variations in Papillary Contour

Normal papillary contour: pyramidal shape

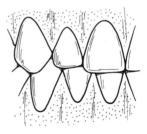

Abnormal contour: bulbous; "overflowing" the embrasure space

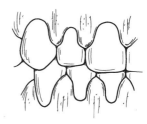

Abnormal contour: missing blunted papillae

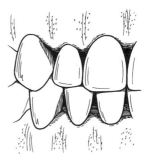

Abnormal contour: crater papillae; "scooped out" appearance

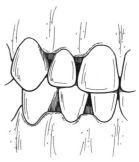

TOOLS FOR PERIODONTAL ASSESSMENT

Tool	Assessment: Natural Dentition	Assessment: Dental Implants
Visual inspection	Gingival color, contour, tone Calculus detection	same
Compressed air	Gingival tone Calculus detection	same
Calibrated probe	**Using metal or plastic probe:** Gingival tone Clinical attachment level Bleeding points Exudate Mucogingival examination Measuring of oral deviations	**Using plastic probe:** Gingival tone Clinical attachment level Bleeding points Exudate

Furcation probe	Furcation involvement	Not applicable (N/A)
Instrument handles	Mobility	Same, using plastic handles
Explorer	Calculus detection Detection of plaque retentive factors and subgingival calculus	N/A
Radiographic	Bone height and density	same

Self-Illuminating Intraoral Mirrors

This illuminated dental mirror combines a disposable front surface mirror with a handpiece containing a 4.75 watt halogen bulb. This illuminated mirror provides high quality light anywhere in the oral cavity, such as the distal surfaces of maxillary molars and lingual surfaces of mandibular anteriors. (Photographs of Denlite mirror courtesy of Welch Allyn WA.)

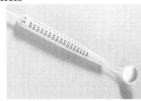

The mirror handpiece also can be used with a tip specifically designed for transillumination of the teeth.

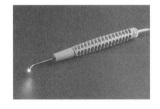

Section 2:

Assessments with Periodontal Probes

TYPES OF PERIODONTAL PROBES

The Periodontal Probe

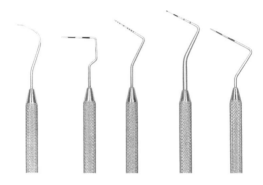

(Courtesy of Hu-Friedy Manufacturing Company.)

The periodontal probe is an instrument of evaluation used in assessing the periodontal health of the tissues. There are two basic types: calibrated and furcation probes.

Periodontal probes have blunt, rod-shaped working ends that are circular or rectangular in cross section. Some designs are marked in millimeter increments and are used for making intraoral measurements. Others, furcation probes, are used to evaluate bone support in the furcation areas of bifurcated and trifurcated teeth.

The Calibrated Periodontal Probe

Findings from an examination with a periodontal probe are an important part of a comprehensive periodontal assessment.

The calibrated periodontal probe is used to

- Determine the consistency of the gingival tissue (i.e., probe is used to apply gentle pressure against the free gingiva)
- Survey sulcus and pockets depths
- Measure clinical attachment levels
- Determine the width of attached gingiva
- Evaluate for presence of bleeding and purulent exudate (i.e., suppuration)

There are many types of probe designs and calibration patterns (i.e., millimeter markings). The calibrated probes pictured here are examples of the many designs available. If you are uncertain of how a probe is calibrated, use a millimeter ruler to determine the millimeter markings.

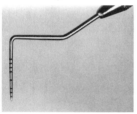

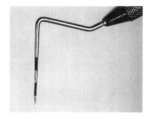

"Traditional" calibrated probe; for ease in reading, there are no marks at the 4 mm or 6 mm reading.

Color coded probes have black bands indicating 1, 2, or 3 mm increments. This particular probe has band markings at 3, 6, 9, and 12 mm.

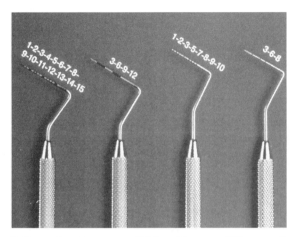

Calibrated probes are available with many different calibration patterns. Examples of some of the probe markings are pictured here. (Courtesy of Hu-Friedy Manufacturing Co., Inc.)

This probe features a right angle–tip design that facilitates adaptation to distal surfaces of molar teeth. (Courtesy of Hu-Friedy Mfg. Co., Inc.)

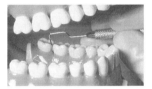

Plastic periodontal probes are used to assess peri-implant tissues. Two examples of plastic probe designs are pictured here.

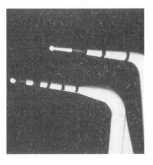

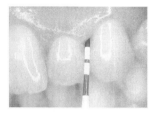

This plastic probe has multicolored markings: green color-coding from 0 to 3 mm, a red mark at 5 mm, and red color-coding from 7 to 10 mm. (Courtesy of Premier Dental Products Co.)

Computerized Probes

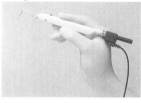

This computer-assisted probe features a lightweight plastic handpiece that is connected to a computer. The handpiece is autoclavable. (Photographs of the computerized probe are courtesy of Florida Probe Corporation.)

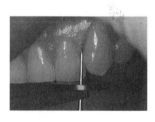

When activated, the metal tip of the computerized probe is inserted into the sulcus or pocket space. The computerized probe is pressure-sensitive and produces a consistent probing force each time it is activated.

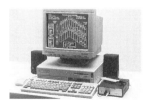

The probe tip is connected to a computer unit that will store information on recession, pocket depth, furcation involvement, suppuration, plaque assessment, and mobility. A paper copy printout of the information can be generated.

PROBING TECHNIQUES

Probing the Distal Surfaces of Maxillary Molars

It is often difficult to position the probe parallel to the distal surface for insertion when probing the distal surfaces of maxillary molars. This problem can be overcome by using an advanced fulcrum and positioning the instrument hand to the side of the patient's face. (Refer to Chapter 7 for information on advanced fulcruming techniques.)

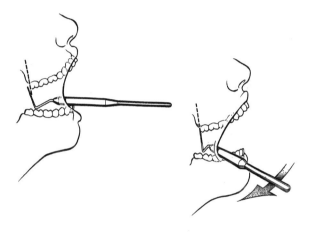

Visual Guidelines for Use of the Probe

Correct Technique: The length of the probe should be held parallel to the long axis of the tooth.

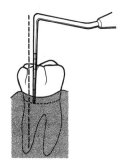

Incorrect Technique: The length of the probe is not parallel to the long axis of the tooth. This error will cause a false reading.

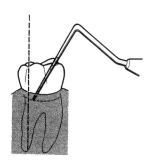

Assessing the Col Area: Visual Guidelines

The interdental col area is an important area to assess because this area is extremely susceptible to disease. It is impossible, however, to obtain a direct reading at the midline of a proximal surface that is in contact with the adjacent tooth. Since the probe cannot be inserted through the contact area, it must be slanted under the contact area.

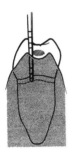

When assessing a proximal surface, walk the probe in small steps, making a mental note of the probe reading at each step. Continue walking the probe interproximally until the working end is touching the contact area.

Slant the working end slightly so that the upper portion tilts away from the contact area and the tip reaches under the contact area. With the probe in this slanted position, gently press downward to touch the attachment area. Take a reading.

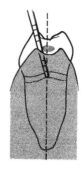

When working from the lingual aspect of the tooth, slant the working end of the probe lingually.

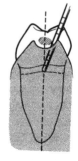

CLINICAL ASSESSMENT USING A PERIODONTAL PROBE

Assessing Pocket Depth

Pocket depth readings are helpful in prescribing home care regimens and educating patients in daily plaque control procedures. For purposes of plaque removal, patients need to understand that a pocket is more difficult to clean and must be aware of the location of pockets in their mouth.

A probing depth is the distance from the <u>gingival margin</u> to the base of the gingival sulcus or pocket as measured with a calibrated periodontal probe.

Assessing Bone Support

In evaluating the periodontal health status of a patient's mouth, it is important to assess the amount of bone support present. Traditional charting techniques have involved the recording of probing depths. Probing depth readings alone, however, provide insufficient data for assessing the bone support. A probing depth is measured in reference to the gingival margin. The probing depth, therefore, is an accurate indicator of bone support <u>only</u> if the gingival margin is at the level of the CEJ.

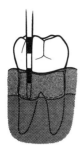
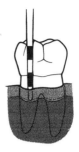

Tooth A: The gingival margin is at the CEJ.

Tooth B: The gingival margin is apical to the CEJ.

The dotted line on these illustrations represents the junctional epithelium on Teeth A and B.

Which tooth has more bone support? Tooth A or Tooth B?

The bone support is approximately equal for Teeth A and B (5 mm).

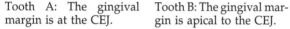

To obtain an accurate clinical picture of bone support, the clinician must assess the bone level in relation to the tooth. Bone support can be accurately noted on a chart by using one of two methods:

1. Record probing depths <u>and</u> the position of the gingival margin. The position of the gingival margin is recorded as a line drawn on an anatomical chart of the dentition. The line must be drawn to accurately represent the millimeters that the gingival margin is coronal or apical to the CEJ.
2. Record clinical attachment level readings. A clinical attachment level is measured in reference to the CEJ, therefore, these readings always accurately reflect the bone level.

A clinical attachment level is the distance from the <u>cementoenamel junction</u> to the base of the gingival sulcus or pocket as measured with a calibrated periodontal probe.

Use of a Calibrated Probe To Determine Clinical Attachment Levels

The position of the gingival margin can change; it moves coronally with edema and apically with recession. The clinical attachment level is measured from the CEJ because it is a fixed point on the tooth that never changes. The bone level can be estimated as being approximately 2 millimeters apical to the junctional epithelium. For example, if the clinical attachment level is 5 mm, then the bone level is approximately 7 mm apical to the CEJ. Clinical attachment level readings, therefore, are important clinical indicators of bone support in an area.

When Gingival Margin is At or Apical To the Cementoenamel Junction

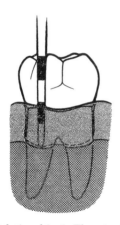 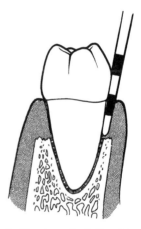

Relationship 1: The gingival margin is approximately level with the CEJ. The dotted line on this illustration represents the junctional epithelium.

A side view of relationship 1, the gingival margin is approximately even with the CEJ. In this case, the clinical attachment level is 5 mm.

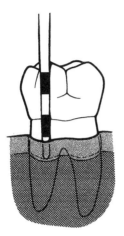 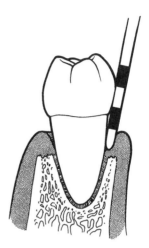

This illustration shows relationship 2 where the gingival margin is apical to the CEJ. When this relationship exists, the CEJ is visible.

This figure shows the side view of the gingival margin apical to the CEJ. In this case, the clinical attachment level is 5 mm.

To determine the clinical attachment level when the <u>gingival margin is at or apical to the CEJ</u>:

1. Determine the level where the CEJ touches the probe.
2. Record the millimeter reading where the probe contacts the CEJ as the clinical attachment level.

When Gingival Margin is Coronal To the Cementoenamel Junction

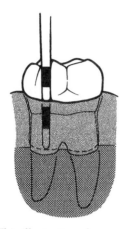 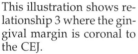 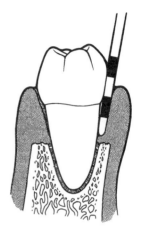

This illustration shows relationship 3 where the gingival margin is coronal to the CEJ.

Side view showing the gingival margin coronal to the CEJ.

Three steps are necessary to determine the clinical attachment level if the gingival margin is coronal to the CEJ:

1. Measure the distance from the gingival margin to the junctional epithelium. This is the *overall measurement.*
2. Determine by tactile sensitivity the location of the CEJ. Measure the distance from the gingival margin to the CEJ. This is the *distance that the margin is coronal to the CEJ.*
3. Subtract the *distance that the margin is coronal to the CEJ* from the *overall measurement.* The difference between these two measurements is the clinical attachment level.

Recording Readings on the Periodontal Chart

For purposes of assessment, each tooth is divided into six areas. Only six readings are recorded per tooth; three readings on the facial aspect and three on the lingual aspect of the tooth. In some cases, the tissue will contact the probe halfway between millimeter marks. Should this occur, the reading is rounded up to the higher millimeter reading. For example, if the reading is at 4.5 mm; the reading should be recorded as 5 mm.

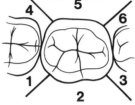

Area 1: distofacial line angle to midline of distal surface
Area 2: facial surface
Area 3: mesiofacial line angle to midline of mesial surface
Area 4: distolingual line angle to midline of distal surface
Area 5: lingual surface
Area 6: mesiolingual line angle to midline of mesial surface

Topography of the Junctional Epithelium

The level of the junctional epithelium is not necessarily uniform around the entire circumference of a tooth. The depths may vary considerably from one spot to the next. For this reason, it is necessary to cover the entire circumference of the tooth with a walking stroke of the probe.

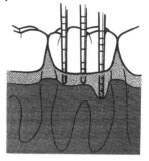

Probing strokes must be close to each other, only approximately 2 mm apart, in order to cover the entire circumference of the sulcus or pocket base with the probe.

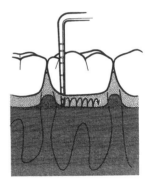

This illustration shows three readings, A, B, C, taken on the facial surface of a mandibular molar. Reading C would be recorded for the facial aspect of this tooth because only a single reading can be recorded per area.

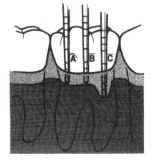

Mucogingival Examination With a Calibrated Probe

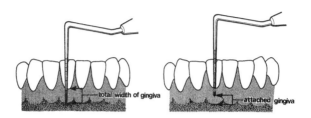

Measuring the width of the attached gingiva

1. On the external surface of the gingiva, measure from the gingival margin to the mucogingival junction. This distance is the *total width of the gingiva.*
2. Insert the probe into the sulcus or pocket and measure the *probing depth* (i.e., the distance from the gingival margin to the junctional epithelium).
3. Subtract the *probing depth* from the *total width of the gingiva,* the difference between these two measurements is the **width of the attached gingiva.**

Use of a Calibrated Probe To Evaluate Oral Deviations

When an oral lesion or deviation is observed in a patient's mouth, the clinician should record this finding on the patient's chart. Information recorded should include the date, size, location, color, and character of the lesion; any information provided by the patient (e.g., duration, sensation, or oral habits) should also be recorded.

A calibrated probe is used in determining the size of the lesion or deviation. It is best to use anatomic references, rather than "length" or "width," to document your measurements (e.g., as the anterior-posterior measurement and the superior-inferior measurement).

Sample chart entry:
January 12, 1997: a soft, red, pedunculated papillary lesion located on buccal mucosa opposite the maxillary left first premolar; measuring 5 mm in an anterior-posterior direction and 6 mm in a superior-inferior direction

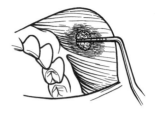

To determine the height of a raised deviation, place the probe tip on normal tissue alongside of the deviation. Imagine a line at the highest part of the deviation, and record this measurement as the height.

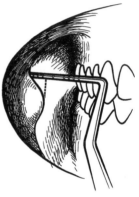

To determine the depth of a sunken deviation, carefully place the probe tip in the deepest part. Imagine a line running from edge to edge of the deviation. The depth is the distance from this imaginary line to the base of the deviation.

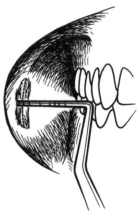

EXAMINING FURCATION AREAS

Furcation involvement occurs when bone loss extends apical to the level where the bifurcation or trifurcation of the root trunk begins and periodontal infection invades the area between and around the roots. Note that this is a classification of the *extent* of furcation involvement. The numerals I, II, III, and IV do not represent millimeter measurements.

CLASSIFICATION OF FURCATION INVOLVEMENT	
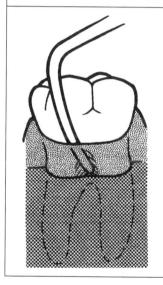	**Class I:** Loss of bone is slight in the furcation area. Furcation concavity can be detected; however, the furcation probe cannot enter the furcation area.

continued

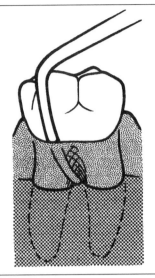

Class II: Partial bone loss in furcation area. Furcation probe will enter the furcation area but not pass through it.

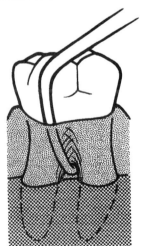

Class III: Complete bone loss in furcation area. Furcation probe will pass between the roots through the entire furcation.

continued

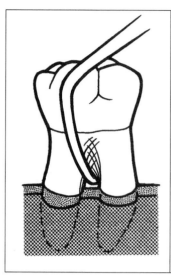

Class IV: Same as Class III except that the furca is visible clinically because of the presence of tissue recession.

ASSESSING FURCATION AREAS

Furcation probes are curved, blunt-tipped instruments used to detect bone loss in the furcation areas of bifurcated and trifurcated teeth.

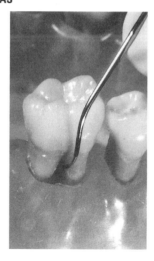

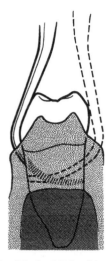 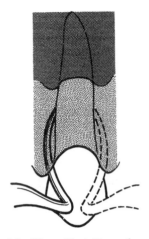

Mandibular Molar (shown here from the proximal, side, view): insert the probe between the mesial and distal roots from the facial and lingual aspect of the tooth.

Maxillary First Premolar (shown here from the facial view): insert the probe between the buccal roots and lingual root from the mesial or distal aspect of tooth.

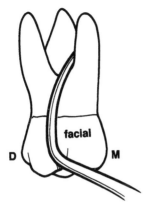

Maxillary Molars (shown from the facial view): insert the probe between the facial and palatal roots from the facial aspect of the tooth.

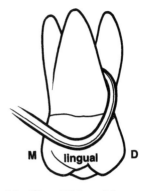

Maxillary Molars (shown from the lingual view): insert the probe between the facial and palatal roots from the disto-lingual, lingual, and mesiolingual on the lingual aspect of the tooth.

ASSESSING MOBILITY AND FREMITUS

Mobility

Mobility refers to the movement a tooth in its socket. Teeth should exhibit slight mobility because of the periodontal ligament. Grade 1, 2, or 3 mobility indicates trauma and/or periodontal pathology.

MOBILITY SCALE:

N = normal physiologic mobility

Grade I = slight mobility, up to 1 mm of horizontal displacement in a facial-lingual direction

Grade II = moderate mobility, greater than 1 mm of displacement in a facial-lingual direction

Grade III = severe mobility, greater than 1 mm of displacement in all directions (i.e., vertical and horizontal)

Technique for Assessing Mobility:

1. Place patient in a normal supine position.
2. Obtain two single-ended instruments with blunt handles. Dry the tooth to be examined.
3. Place the ends of the handles on opposite sides of the tooth (i.e., facial and lingual surfaces).
4. Apply alternating pressure with the handles, first from the facial aspect, then from the lingual. Pathologic mobility is most often evident in a facial-lingual direction.
5. Next, check for vertical mobility by using the end of the instrument handle to exert vertical pressure on the occlusal surface or incisal edge of the tooth.

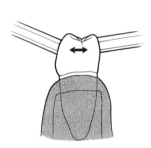 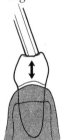

Check for horizontal mobility. Using the ends of two handles, apply alternating pressure, first from the facial and then from the lingual aspect of the tooth.

Check for vertical mobility. Use the end of one handle to exert pressure against the occlusal surface or incisal edge of the tooth.

Fremitus

Fremitus is tooth movement created by the patient's own occlusal force while biting. To assess for fremitus: (1) Place your index finger against the facial surface of a maxillary tooth and ask the patient to tap the teeth together. (2) Feel for vibration (i.e., movement) of the tooth as the patient taps his or her teeth together. (3) Assess each maxillary tooth, in sequence, for fremitus.

FREMITUS SCALE	
First Degree	slight vibrations felt; first-degree fremitus is recorded as "+" on the chart.
Second Degree	definite palpable vibrations; recorded as "++"
Third Degree	clearly visible movement in response to the tapping; recorded as "+++"

ASSESSING DENTAL IMPLANTS

Maintenance therapy for dental implants is similar to a maintenance visit for a patient treated for periodontitis. Peri-implant tissues, however, interact in a different manner from the normal tooth-tissue interface.

The following is a list of objectives for maintenance therapy for dental implants.

1. *Maintenance of alveolar bone support* is evaluated by use of quality radiographs taken with long-cone paralleling technique at specific time intervals. The bone height and density around the implants is compared with previous radiographs of the site.
2. *Control of inflammation*—patient and professional plaque control is important for proper gingival health. Patient home care must be reevaluated and, if necessary, reinforced each time the patient is seen for maintenance. The better the patient performs, the better the possibilities of maintaining stable results.
3. *Maintenance of a healthy and functional implant* includes evaluation of clinical parameters, readjustments, and assessing prosthesis integrity by checking loose screws, cement washout, and material wear; implant, screw, or abutment fracture; unseating of attachments; solder joint wear; implant mobility; and proper adaptation. This phase of maintenance requires consultation with the dentist or specialists in this area.

Peri-implant mucositis is the term used to describe a reversible inflammatory reaction in the soft tissues surrounding a functioning dental implant. The term "peri-implant mucositis" is comparable to gingivitis with the natural dentition.

Peri-implantitis is the term for inflammatory reactions with loss of supporting bone in the tissues surrounding a dental implant.

Osseointegration is the term used to describe the close contact between bone and the implant surface and is a major requirement for implant success. Histologically, the definition of osseointegration is still open for discussion.

Clinically, however, osseointegration corresponds to a dental implant that <u>does NOT present:</u>

- Clinical mobility
- Gingival inflammation of peri-implant tissues
- Discomfort or pain when in function
- Increased clinical attachment levels
- Increased bone loss or radiolucence around the dental implant on radiograph

Peri-implant Probing

Peri-implant probing depths appear to be dependent on the thickness of the mucosa around the abutment. A thicker mucosa generally results in deeper probing depths whereas a keratinized collar around the abutment results in shallower depths. Therefore, the probe reading alone does not necessarily indicate periodontal disease.

In order to interpret probe readings, the clinician must have baseline data relating to the implant; such as, abutment type and size, prosthetic design, the baseline clinical attachment levels, and fixed reference point for probing. Probing measurements must be made from a fixed reference point on the abutment or prosthetic implant crown. Increasing probing readings may indicate a need for tissue evaluation and possible treatment.

Probing should be avoided until postoperative healing is complete, approximately 3 months after abutment connection. Only a light probing technique of approximately 20 grams should be used because the biologic seal is weakly adherent to the abutment. A heavy probing force may be invasive because the probe may penetrate through the biologic seal and could introduce bacteria into the peri-implant environment. Penetration of the plastic probe tip depends on the health (or inflammatory stage of the peri-implant tissues) and the thickness of the mucosa around the abutment.

Clinical examination of the gingival tissue texture, color, and resilience is a subjective indicator of early gingival inflammation. Bleeding upon gentle probing or the presence of exudate provides objective signs of inflammation.

A gentle probing technique with a plastic probe is recommended.

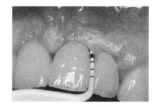

Assessing Implant Mobility

Absence of mobility is an important clinical criteria for dental implants. Visible mobility of an implant after adequate healing time is an indication of peri-implant pathology and failure of the dental implant therapy. Implant mobility is assessed using the same technique as for natural dentition. Instruments with plastic handles should be used to evaluate implant mobility. An absence of mobility is normal.

Implant Failure

The loss of a dental implant may occur a few months after surgical placement or after osseointegration has occurred and the dental implant is in restorative function. Late failures arise from pathological processes that have been classified as disturbances in biomechanical equilibrium (i.e., occlusal overload) and alterations of the host-parasite equilibrium (i.e., infection).

Radiographic image of two dental implants showing lack of complete restorative adaptation.

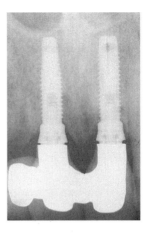

Section 3:

Assessments with Explorers

TYPES OF EXPLORERS

The Dental Explorer

The instrument that provides the best tactile information is the explorer. Explorers are used to locate the following: calculus deposits, tooth surface irregularities, defective margins on restorations, decalcified areas, and carious lesions. Explorers are available in a variety of design types. All design types are not well suited to subgingival use; therefore, the clinician must be knowledgeable about the recommended use of each design type.

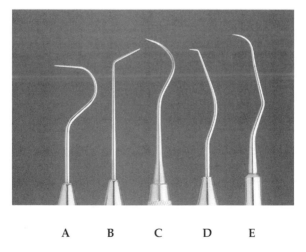

A   B   C   D   E

Explorer types as follows: **A**) Shepherd Hook, **B**) Straight, **C**) Pigtail-type, **D**) Orban-type, and **E**) 11/12-type explorer.

Shepherd Hook and Straight Explorers

Shepherd hook and straight explorers are unpaired explorers. These explorers are limited by short, rigid shanks that reduce tactile conduction. These instruments will not reach much beyond the cementoenamel junction on root surfaces. In addition, the sharp point of these explorers comes in contact with the junctional epithelium when the working end is directed into the gingival crevice. These explorers should be limited to use for detection of dental caries and examination of occlusal surfaces and the surfaces of restorations.

Pigtail and Cowhorn Explorers

The pigtail or cowhorn explorer is a paired explorer with mirror image working ends. This explorer design has two characteristics that limit its use. The short, broadly curved terminal shank causes considerable tissue displacement, limiting its use to normal sulci and shallow pockets. The working end design also restricts the use of this explorer because its sharp point is directed toward the junctional epithelium during subgingival instrumentation. The pigtail or cowhorn explorer is a paired, universal instrument that can be adapted to all anterior and posterior surfaces. These explorers have short functional shanks with a complex design. Pigtail and cowhorn explorers are best when used in normal sulci or shallow pockets extending no deeper than the cervical-third of the root.

Orban-Type Explorers

The Orban-type explorer is an unpaired explorer that has several unique design characteristics. First, the tip of the explorer is bent at a 90° angle to the terminal shank; this design allows the back of the tip to be applied to the pocket base without lacerating the junctional epithelium. The second unique design characteristic of the Orban-type explorer is the straight terminal shank, which allows insertion in a narrow, deep pocket with only slight displacement of the tissue away from the root surface. The straight shank design, however, also limits this explorer to use on anterior teeth and to facial and lingual surfaces of posterior teeth. Adaptation of the tip is difficult on line angles and proximal surfaces of posterior teeth. An Orban-type explorer is an excellent explorer to have available for use in narrow, deep pockets on anterior teeth or facial and lingual surfaces of posterior teeth.

The 11/12-Type Explorer

The 11/12-type explorer is a paired explorer with mirror image working ends. Like the Orban-type explorer, the back of the tip can be applied to the pocket base without lacerating the junctional epithelium. The design characteristic that makes the 11/12-type explorers unique is the shank design. These explorers have long functional shanks with a complex design; thus, these explorers are easily adapted in deep pockets and in areas where access is limited. The 11/12-type explorer is a paired, universal instrument that can be adapted to all anterior and posterior surfaces. The 11/12-type explorer is the most effective explorer design. It adapts well to all surfaces throughout the mouth and is equally useful when exploring near the cementoenamel junction or within 7 mm pockets.

Explorer Design Features

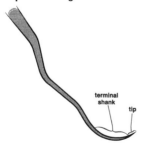

terminal shank

tip

The explorer has a fine, wirelike working end. It is made of flexible metal and is circular in cross section. The working end of an explorer is 1 to 2 mm long and is referred to as its tip.

The actual point of the explorer is never used to assess for calculus or plaque retentive factors; rather, the explorer tip should be adapted to the tooth surface. The explorer tip is used for detection of dental caries.

Explorer Shank Design

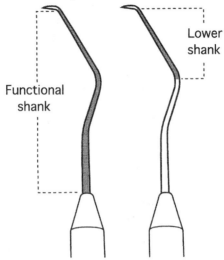

The **functional shank** of an explorer is the portion of the shank from the working end to the final bend, which is next to the instrument handle.

The **lower shank** of an explorer is the section of the shank nearest to the working end. This part of the shank also is termed the **terminal shank.** The lower shank begins below the working end and extends to the first shank bend.

Explorers With Extended Functional Shanks

A comparison of an explorer with a long functional shank on the *left* and an explorer with an extended functional shank on the *right*.

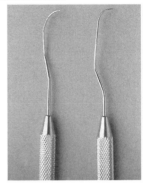

An explorer with extended shank (i.e., After Five 11/12) offers excellent access to proximal pocket defects greater than 5 mm in depth.

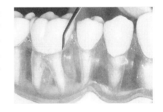

Explorers with extended shanks are helpful when exploring furcation areas located within deep pockets.

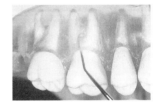

TECHNIQUE FOR USE OF A UNIVERSAL EXPLORER

Selecting the Correct Working End for Anterior Sextants

When using a universal explorer, such as an 11/12-type or a pigtail explorer, you must identify the correct working end. For a particular aspect, one working end is used to instrument the surfaces toward you; the other working end is used to instrument the surfaces away from you. Use these steps to select the correct working end.

Steps for Selecting the Correct Working End for Anterior Sextants

1. Grasp the instrument in a modified pen grasp, and establish a fulcrum.
2. Place either working end on the tooth surface on which you wish to work.
3. Hold the instrument so that the handle is parallel to the long axis of the tooth surface.
4. Look closely at the working end that is adapted against the tooth surface. If the tip curves toward the tooth, this is the correct working end for this tooth surface.

RULE: For anterior teeth, the *tip* of the working end should curve *toward* the tooth.

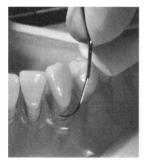

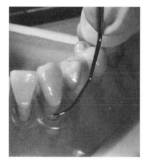

Correct: Tip curves toward surface on which you plan to work when handle is parallel to tooth surface.

Incorrect: Tip curves away from surface on which you plan to work when handle is parallel to tooth surface.

Use of a Universal Explorer On Anterior Tooth Surfaces

Example: Mandibular anteriors—facial aspect with 11/12-Type Explorer

The step-by-step approach to using a universal explorer on anterior teeth is shown for the facial aspect of the mandibular anteriors. The surfaces being instrumented are, for a right-handed clinician, the surfaces toward you; or for a left-handed clinician, the surfaces away from you. Assessment of the remaining surfaces of the mandibular anteriors and of the maxillary anteriors is performed in a similar manner.

Select the correct working end for use on the facial aspect of the mandibular left canine, working from the midline of the facial and onto the mesial surface. Adapt the tip (not the point) of the explorer to the tooth surface. Activate a feather-light assessment stroke.

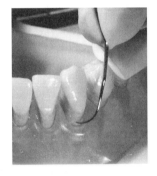

Relax your grasp. Roll the instrument handle to adapt the explorer tip to the next area. Establish correct angulation, and activate a sweeping stroke.

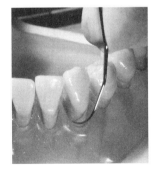

Roll the instrument handle to obtain proper adaptation to the mesiofacial line angle. Establish correct angulation and activate a stroke.

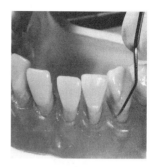

Relax your grasp, and roll the instrument handle to adapt to the mesial surface. Adapt the explorer tip, and activate a stroke.

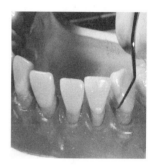

Continue strokes until you have assessed at least 50% of mesial proximal surface from the facial aspect. The other 50% of the mesial surface will be assessed when you instrument the lingual aspect with the explorer.

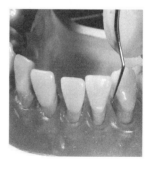

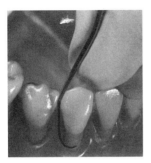

Work across the sextant, ending with the distal surface of the right canine. Change operator positions and complete the other 50% of the facial aspect, beginning with the mesial surface of the right canine.

Selecting the Correct Working End for Posterior Sextants

When using a paired universal explorer, you must identify the correct working end for use on a particular aspect of the tooth. One working end is used to instrument the **facial aspect** of a sextant; the other working end is used to instrument the **lingual aspect** of the sextant. Use these steps to select the working end on the facial or lingual aspect.

Steps for Selecting the Correct Working End: A Paired Universal Explorer.

1. Grasp the instrument in a modified pen grasp, and establish a fulcrum.
2. Place either working end on a proximal surface apical to the contact area. Establish an appropriate finger rest. Position the handle so that it is as parallel as possible to the long axis of the tooth.
3. Look closely at the **shank nearest the working end**: if the lower shank **is parallel with** the proximal surface, this is the **correct** working end for this aspect.

> **RULE: For posterior teeth, the lower shank should be parallel to the proximal surface.**

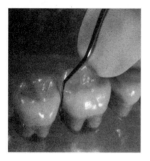

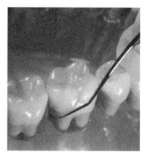

Correct: If the lower shank is parallel with the proximal surface, this is the correct working end for this aspect.

Incorrect: If the lower shank crosses the facial or lingual surface in an oblique manner, this is the incorrect working end for this aspect.

Use of a Paired Universal Explorer on Posterior Tooth Surfaces

Example: Mandibular Right Posteriors, *Facial Aspect* with an 11/12-Type Explorer

The step-by-step approach to using a universal explorer on posterior teeth is shown for the mandibular right posterior teeth, facial aspect. The lingual aspect of this sextant is completed in a similar manner. The same sequencing of instrumentation is used with the remaining three posterior sextants.

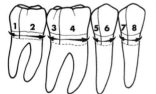

1. The tooth surfaces of the facial aspect should be completed in the order shown in this illustration.

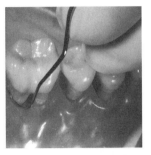

2. Begin with the last molar in the sextant. Adapt the leading third of the tip to the distofacial line angle. The tip of the working end should point toward the back of the mouth because this is the direction in which you are working.

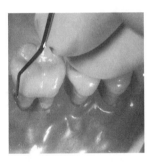

3. Work across the distal surface with flowing light strokes. The strokes should overlap one another.

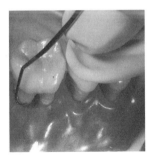

4. While maintaining your fulcrum, lift the working end away from the tooth and turn it so that the tip "points" forward, toward the front of the mouth. Reposition the tip at the distofacial line angle. Activate an oblique working stroke.

5. Work across the facial surface, using a series of oblique strokes. As you approach the furcation, roll the instrument handle to maintain adaptation of the explorer tip.

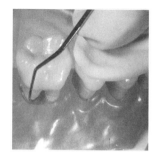

6. Turn the explorer tip, and adapt it to the distal surface of the mesial root within the furcation area.

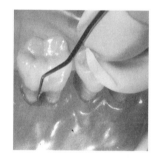

7. Explore the mesial half of the mesial root.

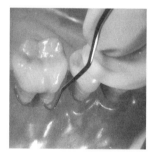

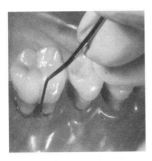

8. Roll the instrument handle to maintain adaptation as you work onto the mesial surface of the tooth.

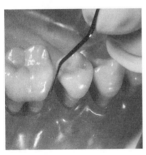

9. Continue strokes until you have instrumented at least 50% of the mesial surface from the facial aspect. The other 50% of the mesial surface will be assessed from the lingual aspect.

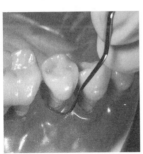

10. Move onto the next tooth in the sextant. Begin at the distofacial line angle, and work onto the distal surface.

INTERPRETATION OF SUBGINGIVAL CONDITIONS

The ability to interpret what you are feeling subgingivally with an explorer is an important skill that takes time and concentration to develop. The following descriptions from an article by Dr. J. Richard Trott should aid you in acquiring the technique of interpreting what you feel.*

Normal Conditions

Your fingers do not feel any interruptions in the path of the explorer when it is inserted and withdrawn from the gingival crevice.

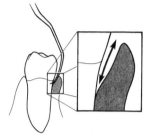

Large Subgingival Calculus Deposit

The explorer moves over the tooth surface, encounters the raised deposit, moves over it, and returns down to the tooth surface. This can be compared to the sensation of roller skating over speed bumps in a parking lot.

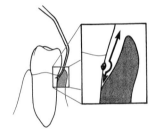

Granular Subgingival Calculus Deposits

There is a gritty sensation as the explorer passes over fine, granular calculus deposits. This is similar to the sensation experienced when roller skating over a gravel surface.

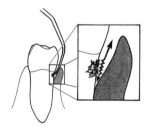

*Trott, J.R.: The cross subgingival calculus explorer. Dent Digest 67:481-3, 1961.

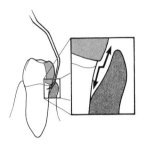

Overhanging Margin of a Restoration

The explorer passes over the surface of the restoration and suddenly dips onto the tooth surface. This condition can be distinguished because the explorer "dips in" rather than moving up and around as for a calculus deposit. This can be compared to skating over a section of a road that has large potholes.

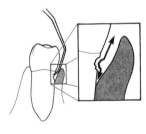

Carious Lesion

The explorer dips in and then comes out again to proceed along the tooth surface. The sunken area of the carious lesion will be irregular. The base of the lesion usually is soft and can be penetrated with the point of the explorer. This would be like skating into a pothole that had just been repaired with asphalt. The skate blades would sink into the partially hardened asphalt.

MECHANIC'S CHECK: COMMON CAUSES OF UNDETECTED CALCULUS

Location of Undetected Calculus Deposits	Technique Error
No particular pattern to the location of undetected deposits	• Use of inappropriate explorer design for the task • Grasp too tight, choking grasp • Middle finger not on shank; fewer vibrations can be felt through the instrument handle • Middle finger applied firmly against shank rather than resting lightly on shank; firm pressure against shank reduces tactile sensitivity • Failure to overlap assessment strokes; some portions of the tooth surface were not explored
Undetected deposits on line angles or midlines of teeth	• Failure to overlap strokes in these areas • Not using rolling handle to maintain adaptation at line angles • Not using circumferential strokes in these areas
Undetected deposits on proximal surfaces of teeth	• Strokes not extended apical to contact area; at least 50% of each proximal surface should be explored from the facial and lingual aspects of the tooth • Failure to insert explorer to the base of the gingival crevice in the proximal area before initiating strokes in a coronal direction

continued

Location of Undetected Calculus Deposits	Technique Error
Undetected deposits near the junctional epithelium	• Failure to insert explorer to the base of the gingival crevice before initiating stroke in a coronal direction

USE OF AN EXPLORER FOR CARIES DETECTION

Instrument Selection

An explorer for caries detection should have a strong rigid shank to withstand a force applied against the tooth surface. A straight or Shepherd Hook explorer is a good choice for caries detection. The tip of an 11/12-type or a pigtail explorer can be damaged if used for caries detection. Once damaged, the burred working end will not provide accurate tactile information to the clinician's fingers for detection of calculus.

Types of Carious Lesions

- Enamel caries occur in *pits and fissures* of lingual surfaces near the cingulum of anterior teeth and on the occlusal surfaces and buccal pits of posterior teeth.
- *Smooth surface enamel caries* can occur on the facial, lingual, and proximal aspects of the crown.
- *Root surface caries* occur on root surfaces that are exposed because of tissue recession. Root surface caries also are common findings within periodontal pockets where apical migration of the junctional epithelium exposes the root surface to the oral environment. This type of caries is most commonly seen in geriatric patients.
- *Recurrent decay* occurs along the margins of restorations.

Caries Detection

Enamel caries often can be detected visually by changes in the appearance of the enamel. The lesion may appear chalky-white, gray, brown, or black in color. When pressure is applied with the explorer tip against the walls of the lesion, the surface will feel soft and the point can be felt to penetrate or "catch in" the surface of the lesion. Subgingivally, a smooth surface lesion will be detected as a rough, concave area on the surface of the root.

TECHNIQUE FOR CARIES DETECTION

The general technique for caries detection is to apply light pressure with the point of the explorer against the region of suspected caries.

1. **Pit and Fissure Caries.** Direct the point straight into the pit or fissure, and apply light pressure. Trace the entire length of a fissure with the explorer while applying light pressure downward into the developmental depression. If caries is present, the tip will penetrate or "catch" in the surface of the enamel.
2. **Smooth Surface Caries.** Move the tip of the explorer over the enamel or root surface, be alert for roughness, discontinuity, or change in hardness of the tooth surface. Visually, check for discoloration of enamel surfaces.
3. **Root Surface Caries.** While assessing the root surface, you will feel the explorer dip in and then come out again as it proceeds along the surface of the root. The depressed area of caries will feel rough and can be penetrated by the point of the explorer.
4. **Recurrent Decay.** Trace the margin of the restoration with the point of the explorer. If recurrent decay is present, you may be able to penetrate the tooth surface adjacent to the margin of the restoration.

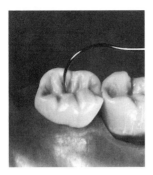

On occlusal surfaces, position the working end of the explorer so that the point can be applied straight into the pit or fissure.

Section 4:

Periodontal Screening and Recording System

The American Dental Association and the American Academy of Periodontology suggest that routine dental examinations include the Periodontal Screening and Recording (PSR) system. The PSR is an efficient easy-to-use system for the detection of periodontal disease.

A specially designed periodontal probe is used with the PSR.

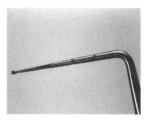

- It has a ball-tipped end; the ball is 0.5 mm in diameter and is designed to minimize trauma to the junctional epithelium.
- The probe is color-coded with a band extending from 3.5 mm to 5.5 mm.

The periodontal probe is inserted into the sulcus or pocket and gently walked around the circumference of each natural tooth or implant using the same probing technique as for a comprehensive periodontal examination.

The unique aspects of the PSR screening are the manner in which the probe is read and the minimal amount of information recorded. Instead of reading and recording millimeter readings, for the PSR, the clinician only needs to observe the position of the colored band in relation to the gingival margin and the presence of furcation invasion, mobility, mucogingival problems, or recession.

Only one score is recorded for each sextant in the mouth. In each sextant, only the highest code obtained is recorded. An "X" is recorded if a sextant is edentulous.

PSR Codes

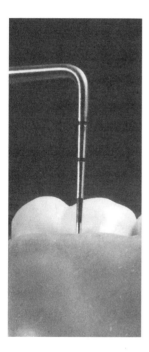

CODE 0:
Colored band is completely visible in the deepest sulcus or pocket in the sextant.

No calculus or defective margins are detected.

Gingival tissues are healthy with no bleeding evident upon gentle probing.

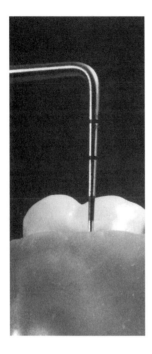

CODE 1:
Colored band is completely visible in the deepest sulcus or pocket in the sextant.

No calculus or defective margins are detected.

Bleeding is event with gentle probing.

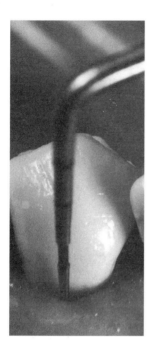

CODE 2:
Colored band is completely visible in the deepest sulcus or pocket in the sextant.

Supra- or subgingival calculus or defective margins are detected.

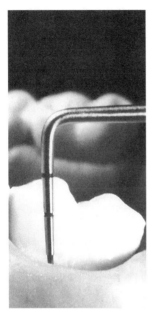

CODE 3:
Colored band is partially visible in the deepest sulcus or pocket in the sextant.

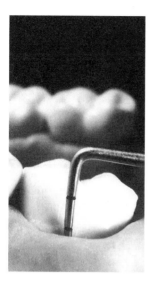

CODE 4:
Colored band is not visible in the deepest sulcus or pocket in the sextant. This indicates a probing depth of greater than 5.5 mm.

CODE *
The * symbol is added to any sextant exhibiting any of the following abnormalities:

- Furcation invasion
- Mobility
- Mucogingival problems
- Recession extending into the colored band

Recording PSR Codes in the Patient's Chart

The PSR code is recorded in a box chart.

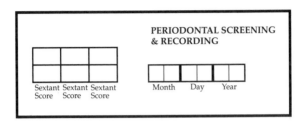

For example, the box chart would look like the one below for a PSR completed on May 14, 1997, with the following scores:

Max. right posterior sextant = Code 3
Max. anterior sextant = Code 2
Max. left posterior sextant = Code 1
Mand. right posterior sextant = Code 3
Mand. anterior sextant = Code 3
Mand. left posterior sextant = Code 4, with furcation invasion and mobility present

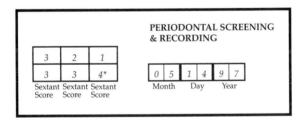

Implications of PSR Codes for Patient Management

CODE 0:   Reinforce daily plaque control habits.

CODE 1:   Reinforce daily plaque control habits. Provide appropriate treatment, including debridement of subgingival plaque.

CODE 2:   Reinforce daily plaque control habits. Provide appropriate treatment, including debridement of subgingival plaque, supra- and subgingival calculus, and correction of plaque-retentive margins of restorations.

CODE 3:   If a single sextant scores a Code 3, a comprehensive periodontal examination is indicated for that sextant. A comprehensive examination should include probing depths (6 reading per tooth), gingival recession, mobility, mucogingival problems, furcation invasions, and appropriate radiographs.

If two or more sextants score Code 3, a comprehensive periodontal examination is indicated for the entire mouth.

CODE 4:   Perform a comprehensive periodontal examination and charting of the entire mouth.

CODE *:   If an abnormality is present in a sextant with a Code 0, 1, or 2 score, note the abnormality.

If an abnormality is present in a sextant with a Code 3 or 4 score, perform a comprehensive periodontal examination and charting of the entire mouth.

Section 5:

Communicating Findings to Patients—Intraoral Imaging Systems

Intraoral imaging systems are quickly becoming commonplace in today's modern dental practices. The pen-sized camera combined with a computer screen is used to show patients problems that they otherwise could not see. Dentists and hygienists are reporting that intraoral imaging improves patient communication and acceptance of treatment plans.

Intraoral imaging systems are helpful in:

- Improving communication between the dental healthcare provider and patient
- Improved patient understanding of the need for treatment
- Documentation of pre- and posttreatment conditions, in the form of "before and after" photographs
- Documentation of intraoral conditions and lesions

Intraoral imaging systems are one example of the use of advanced technology in the dental office. Pictured here is the Reveal SRL system from Welch Allyn.

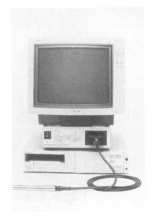

Section 6:

References and Suggested Readings

Beck, J.D.: Periodontal implications: Older adults. Ann Periodontol Nov;1(1):322-57, 1996.

Beck, J.D., Slade, G.D.: Epidemiology of periodontal diseases. Curr Opin Periodontol 3:3-9, 1996.

Beck, J.D., Koch, G.G., Offenbacher, S.: Incidence of attachment loss over 3 years in older adults—new and progressing lesions. Community Dent Oral Epidemiol Oct;23(5):291-6, 1995.

Beck, J.D.: Methods of assessing risk for periodontitis and developing multi-factorial models. J Periodontol May;65(5 Suppl):468-78, 1994.

Beck, J.D.: The epidemiology of root surface caries: North American studies. Adv Dent Res Jul;7(1):42-51, 1993.

Breen, H.J., Rogers, P.A., Slaney, R.E., Lawless, H,C., Austin, J.S., Gillett, I.R., Johnson, N.W.: Option-4 algorithm for automated disc probe: reduction in the variance of site-specific relative attachment level measurements. J Periodontol May;68(5):456-66, 1997.

Breen, H.J., Rogers, P.A., Lawless, H,C., Austin, J.S., Johnson, N.W.: Important differences in clinical data from third, second, and first generation periodontal probes. J Periodontol Apr;68(4):335-45, 1997.

Chapple, I.L: Periodontal disease diagnosis: current status and future developments. J Dent Jan;25(1):3-15, 1997.

Christensen, G.J.: Intraoral television cameras: Presenting a major new use. J Am Dent Assoc 125:439-42, 1994.

Claffey, N., Kelly, A., Bergquist, J., Egelberg, J.: Patterns of attachment loss in advanced periodontitis patients monitored following initial periodontal treatment. J Clin Periodontol Jun;23(6):523-31, 1996.

Claffey, N., Egelberg, J.: Clinical indicators of probing attachment loss following initial periodontal treatment in advanced periodontitis patients. J Clin Periodontol Sep;22(9):690-6, 1995.

Davis, T.: PSR offers quick, easy periodontal screening. J Can Dent Assoc Sep;61(9):770, 1995.

Drake, C.W., Beck, J.D., Lawrence, H.P., Koch, G.G.: Three-year coronal caries incidence and risk factors in North Carolina elderly. Caries Res;31(1):1-7, 1997.

Farr, C.: Smarter perio: New technologies add intelligence, speed and accuracy to diagnosis and treatment. Dentistry Today Oct;78-80, 1995.

Freed, J.R., Perry, D.A., Kushman, J.E.: Aspects of quality of dental hygiene care in supervised and unsupervised practices. J Public Health Dent Spring;57(2):68-75, 1997.

Hujoel, P.P., Makinen, K.K., Bennett, C.B., Isokangas, P.J., Isotupa, K.P., Pape, H.R. Jr., Lamont, R.J., DeRouen, T.A., Davis, S.: Do caries explorers transmit infections with persons? An evaluation of second molar caries onsets. Caries Res 29(6):461-6, 1995.

Khocht, A., Zohn, H., Deasy, M., Chang, K.M.: Assessment of periodontal status with PSR and traditional clinical periodontal examination. J Am Dent Assoc Dec;126(12):1658-65, 1995.

Magnusson, I., Lindhe, J.: Current concepts in diagnosis and treatment of periodontitis. Semin Orthod Mar;2(1):13-20, 1996.

Nasi, J.H.: Background to, and implementation of, the Periodontal Screening and Recording (PSR) procedure in the USA. Int Dent J Oct;44(5 Suppl 1):585-8, 1994.

O'Reilly, P.G., Claffey, N.M.: Identifying losing sites at periodontal reevaluation. Curr Opin Periodontol 3:68-77, 1996.

Piazzini, L.F.: Periodontal screening & recording (PSR) application in children and adolescent. J Clin Pediatr Dent Spring;18(3):165-71, 1994.

Rams, T.E., Slots, J.: Comparison of two pressure-sensitive periodontal probes and a manual periodontal probe in shallow and deep pockets. Int J Periodontics Restorative Dent Dec;13(6):520-9, 1993.

Ship, J.A., Beck, J.D.: Ten-year longitudinal study of periodontal attachment loss in healthy adults. Oral Surg Oral Med Oral Pathol Oral Radiol Endod Mar;81(3):281-90, 1996.

Tomlinson, J.O.: Explore the possibilities with a new high-tech trend: Intraoral imaging systems. Practical Hygiene May/Jun;3(3):23-27, 1995.

Villata L., Baelum V.: Reproducibility of attachment level recordings using an electronic and a conventional probe. J Periodontol Dec;67(12):1292-300, 1996.

Williams, R.C., Beck, J.D., Offenbacher, S.N.: The impact of new technologies to diagnose and treat periodontal disease. A look to the future. J Clin Periodontol Mar;23(3 Pt 2):299-305, 1996.

3

Introduction to
Periodontal Debridement

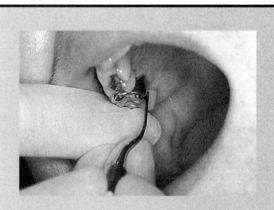

In this chapter

Section 3:

Classifications of Hand-Activated Instruments

- Sickle Scalers
- Periodontal Files
- Curets: Universal and Area-Specific Designs

Section 4:

Analysis of Instrument Design Features

- Sickle Scalers
- Universal Curets
- Area-Specific Curets

Section 5:

References and Suggested Readings

Section 1:

Periodontal Debridement: A New Treatment Paradigm for Periodontal Instrumentation

Recent research findings have stimulated a paradigm shift in the non-surgical treatment of periodontal disease. The current treatment paradigm recognizes that periodontal disease occurs when bacterial flora overwhelm the host's immune response. Emphasis is on the treatment of tissue inflammation to achieve periodontal healing and repair. The goal is returning the tissue to a healthy, non-inflamed state that can be maintained by the patient. Consideration is given to host response factors, such as medications, smoking, neutrophil deficiencies, and systemic illness.

Periodontal debridement is the emerging paradigm for non-surgical treatment of periodontal disease, and scaling and root planing represent the old treatment paradigm. "Scaling" and "root planing" are the traditional terms used to describe the mechanical removal of calculus and diseased hard tissues. The emphasis of scaling and root planing has been root smoothness accomplished by intentional cementum removal. In contrast, the emphasis of periodontal debridement is control of bacterial plaque and plaque retentive calculus and obtaining a favorable tissue response. **Iatrogenic damage** is damage as the result of professional treatment (e.g., damage to the tooth surface as the result of periodontal instrumentation). Periodontal debridement strives to achieve tissue healing with minimal iatrogenic damage to the soft tissue and cementum.

TERMINOLOGY

Scaling and root planing were traditionally defined as the removal of calculus deposits from coronal and root surfaces and the planing to smoothness of the root surface. Root planing traditionally has included the aggressive removal of cementum; for this reason, this book will use the term ''debridement'' instead of ''scaling and root planing.''

Periodontal debridement is the removal or disruption of bacterial plaque, its byproducts, and plaque retentive calculus deposits from coronal surfaces, root surfaces, and within the sulcus or pocket space as indicated for the periodontal healing and repair. Conservation of cementum is a goal of periodontal debridement.

- **Coronal debridement** is the mechanical removal of bacterial plaque and plaque retentive calculus deposits from coronal tooth surfaces.
- **Root surface debridement** is the mechanical removal of bacterial plaque, its byproducts, and plaque retentive calculus deposits from root surfaces.
- **Deplaquing** is the mechanical disruption of subgingival bacterial plaque and its byproducts from the sulcus or pocket space.

COMPARISON OF OLD AND NEW TREATMENT PARADIGMS FOR INSTRUMENTATION

	Old Paradigm	New Paradigm
Focus	Calculus removal and smooth root surfaces	Tissue healing and repair Removal of bacterial plaque, endotoxin, and plaque retentive calculus with minimal iatrogenic damage to the tooth to achieve periodontal healing Total calculus removal is not attainable; soft tissue healing has been demonstrated despite the presence of calculus.
Root Surfaces	Endotoxins were thought to be absorbed into the surface of the cementum or tightly bound to cementum. Therefore, cementum must be removed. Cementum removal was intentional. Extensive instrumentation removed significant amounts of cementum.	Current research indicates that endotoxins are loosely adherent and are easily removed by washing or light instrumentation strokes. Conservation of cementum is a goal. Cementum removal is damaging to the periodontium. Thorough deplaqueing of root surfaces is indicated. Unattached plaque can be flushed from the sulcus or pocket by the fluid lavage produced by mechanized ultrasonic or sonic instruments.

continued

	Old Paradigm	New Paradigm
Method	Hand-activated instrumentation is preferred.	A combination of hand-activated and ultrasonic instrumentation is preferred.
Success	Calculus removal and attainment of smooth root surfaces.	Periodontal healing and repair
Concepts	1. All calculus must be removed before healing can occur. 2. Endotoxins are absorbed into the cementum, thus altering the cementum. 3. Removal of cementum is necessary for tissue healing.	1. Tissue healing can occur in the presence of residual calculus. The clinician should re-evaluate the healing response after initial therapy and proceed as indicated. 2. Endotoxins are easily removed from the surface of the cementum. 3. Cementum should be conserved.

Section 2:

Design of Hand-Activated Instruments

INSTRUMENT BALANCE

An instrument that is not balanced will be more difficult to use and can result in stress to the clinician's hand and arm muscles. An instrument is *balanced* if the working ends are centered on an imaginary line running through the long axis of the handle. An easy way to determine if an instrument is balanced is to place the instrument on a line of a lined writing tablet. Align the midline of the handle with the line on the paper; the instrument is balanced if the working ends fall on the same line as the midline of the handle.

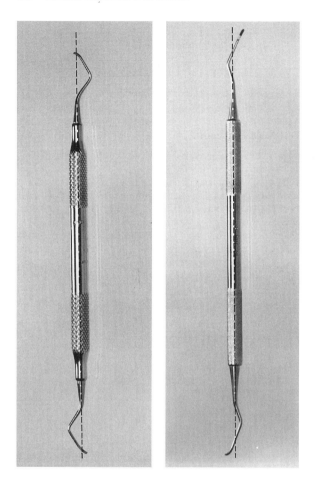

The instrument shown above on the left is balanced. The instrument shown above on the right is not balanced.

DESIGN FEATURES OF INSTRUMENT SHANKS

The instrument shank is an extension device that increases the length of the instrument so that the working end can be placed on the tooth root.

Simple Shank Design

The shank of a periodontal instrument usually has **bends** in one or more places. A shank that is bent in one plane has a simple shank design. A shank that is bent in two planes has a complex shank design.

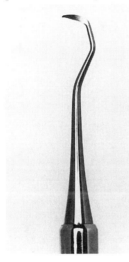

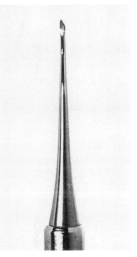

Instrument A, side view. When viewed from the side, it bends from front-to-back.

Instrument A, front view. When viewed from the front, the shank appears to be straight. Instrument A, therefore, has a simple shank design.

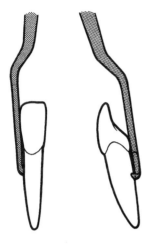

Instruments with simple shanks are used on anterior teeth. The crowns of anterior teeth are wedge-shaped. An instrument with a simple shank will reach along the crown and onto the root surface.

Complex Shank Design

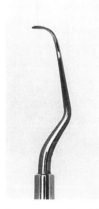

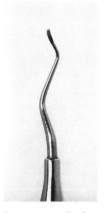

Instrument B, side view. The shank is bent from front-to-back.

Instrument B, front view. The shank also is bent from side-to-side. Instrument B, therefore, has a complex shank.

The crowns of posterior teeth are rounded and over-hang their roots. An instrument with a complex shank is needed to reach around the crown and onto the root surface. Complex shank designs were developed to allow subgingival instrumentation of posterior teeth.

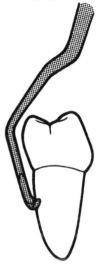 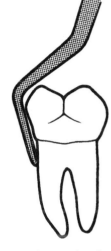

The front-to-back bends allow access to buccal and lingual aspects of the root.

The side-to-side bends allow access to the proximal (i.e., mesial and distal) aspects of the root.

The Functional and Lower Shank

The functional shank is the portion of the shank from the working end to the final bend, next to the instrument handle.

The lower shank is the section of the shank nearest to the working end. This part of the shank also is called the terminal shank. The lower shank begins below the working end and extends to the first shank bend.

The working ends of instruments with short functional shanks can be used to reach the coronal surfaces
of the teeth. The working ends of instruments with long
functional shanks can be used to reach the coronal and
root surfaces of the teeth.

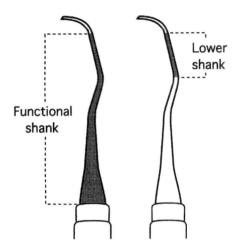

The shaded area on the instrument to the left indicates
the **functional shank.** The shaded area on the instrument
on the right indicates the **lower or terminal shank.**

Shank Flexibility

Instrument shanks may be flexible, moderately flexible,
or rigid in design. The function of a particular instrument
determines how much flexibility is desirable. Instruments designed to fracture large calculus deposits from
the tooth require strong, rigid shanks. Instruments designed to locate small deposits beneath the gingival margin require flexible shanks.

Flexible shanks are used to enhance tactile information to the clinician's hands. Visual information is of
limited use during subgingival instrumentation. Instead,
the clinician relies on his or her sense of touch to locate

irregularities on the root surface. Vibrations are created as the working end is displaced while moving over irregularities on the tooth surface. These vibrations are transmitted from the working end, through the shank, and into the handle. The clinician feels the vibrations with his or her fingers as they rest on the shank and handle.

Shank Type	Characteristics	Intended Use
Flexible	Shank will yield as the working end encounters rough surfaces or deposits. This type provides the most tactile information to the clinician's fingers.	For detection and removal of subgingival calculus deposits Examples: explorers, area-specific curets
Moderately Flexible	Shank will yield slightly as the working end encounters rough surfaces or deposits. This type provides some tactile information to the clinician's fingers.	For removal of medium-sized or small deposits of calculus Example: universal curets
Rigid	Shank will withstand strong forces applied during calculus removal. This type provides limited tactile information to the clinician's fingers.	For removal of large-sized deposits of calculus Examples: sickle scalers, periodontal files

DESIGN AND INSTRUMENT USE

In order to determine the intended use of any instrument, first consider the classification of the working end in combination with the shank design.

Working End	Use
Explorer	Assessment of root surfaces
Sickle scaler	Removal of large-sized supragingival calculus deposits
Universal curet	Removal of medium- and small-sized supra- and subgingival calculus deposits
Area-specific curet	Removal of small supra- and subgingival calculus and endotoxins

Next, consider the design characteristics of the shank.

Shank Design	Surfaces
Short functional shank	Coronal surfaces
Long functional shank	Coronal and root surfaces
Simple shank bends	Anterior teeth
Complex shank bends	Posterior teeth

Suppose that an instrument is a sickle scaler with a short complex shank design. This instrument would be used to remove large deposits from the coronal surfaces of posterior teeth.

A universal curet with a long complex shank would be used to remove light to medium deposits from coronal and root surfaces of posterior teeth.

An area-specific curet with a long simple shank would be used to remove light deposits and endotoxins from the coronal and root surfaces of anterior teeth.

Section 3:

Classifications of Hand-Activated Instruments

SICKLE SCALERS

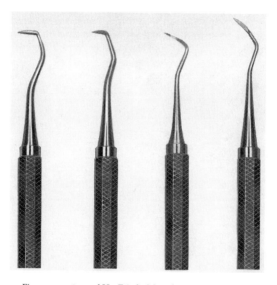

Figures courtesy of Hu-Friedy Manufacturing Company.

Sickle scalers are used to remove large calculus deposits from enamel surfaces. The design features of these instruments restrict them to use on enamel surfaces. Direct application to the root surface would most likely result in excessive removal of cementum from the root surface. Designs are limited to use on either the anterior or posterior teeth.

DESIGN CHARACTERISTICS OF SICKLE SCALERS	
Lateral surfaces	Straight; meet in a pointed tip
Relationship of face to shank	Face at a 90° angle to lower shank
Number of cutting edges	2 cutting edges per working end
Working end in cross-section	Triangular
Functional shank	Short, rigid
Application to sextants and surfaces	Anterior designs limited to use on anterior teeth; posterior designs limited to use on posterior teeth
Use on crown and root surfaces	Limited to use on enamel tooth surfaces

Examples of anterior sickle scalers include the OD-1, Jacquette-30, Jacquette-33, Whiteside-2, USC-128, Towner-U15, Goldman-H6, and Goldman-H7. Posterior sickle scalers have two paired working ends. The paired working ends are mirror-images of one another. For example the Jacquette 34 working end is paired with the Jacquette 35 working end; the Jacquette 34 is a mirror-image of the Jacquette 35. Both of these working ends are needed to debride all the tooth surfaces of a posterior sextant (i.e., mesial, distal, facial, and lingual). The paired working ends of a posterior sickle scaler may be found on two single-ended instruments or may be combined on one double-ended instrument. In addition to the Jacquette 34/35, examples of paired posterior sickle scalers include: Jacquette 14/15; Jacquette 31/32; Ball 2/3; Mecca 11/12; and Catatonia 107/108.

PERIODONTAL FILES

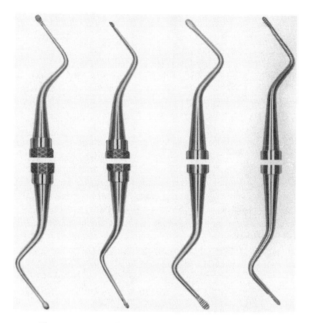

Figures courtesy of Hu-Friedy Manufacturing Company.

Periodontal files are used to prepare calculus deposits before removal with another instrument. There are two instances when periodontal files can facilitate calculus removal. The first instance is the removal of a burnished calculus deposit. Normally, the outer layer of a calculus deposit is rough because of its layer-by-layer formation. A burnished calculus deposit is one in which the outer most layer of calculus is removed rather than the entire deposit. The remaining calculus deposit will have a smooth outer surface. Burnishing usually results from a cutting edge-to-tooth surface angulation of less than a 45° angle. Once burnished, a deposit is difficult to remove because the cutting edge tends to slide over the smooth outer surface. Removal of a burnished calculus deposit is facilitated by using a periodontal file to scratch or roughen the deposit. The roughened deposit can then be removed with another instrument. Periodontal files also can be used to crush a calculus deposit to facilitate removal with another hand-activated instrument.

The design features of periodontal files restrict them to use on enamel surfaces or application to the outer surface of subgingival calculus deposits. Direct application to the root surface would most likely result in excessive removal of cementum from the root surface. Designs are limited to use on the anterior or posterior teeth. Examples of periodontal files include: Organ 10/11, Organ 12/13, Hirschfeld 3/7, Hirschfeld 5/11, and Hirschfeld 9/10.

DESIGN CHARACTERISTICS OF PERIODONTAL FILES

Working end	Working end is thin in width and is rounded, rectangular, or oblong-shaped
Cutting edges	Straight
Number of cutting edges	Multiple
Relationship of cutting edges to shank	90° to 105°
Functional shank	Rigid shank
Application to sextants and surfaces	Instrument designed for use on mesial and distal surfaces or on facial and lingual surfaces; each working end is designed for single-surface application
Use on crown and root surfaces	Limited to use on enamel surfaces or application to outer surface of calculus deposits

CURETS: UNIVERSAL AND AREA-SPECIFIC DESIGNS

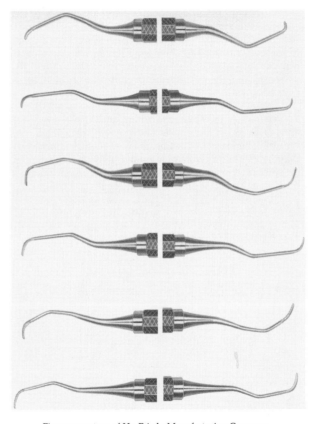

Figures courtesy of Hu-Friedy Manufacturing Company.

Universal Curets

Universal curets are used to remove light or medium supragingival and subgingival calculus deposits from enamel and cemental tooth surfaces. These instruments have functional shanks of intermediate length for access to the cervical-third of the root. The name "universal" reflects the fact that a universal curet can be applied to all tooth surfaces in the anterior and posterior sextants of the mouth.

Like posterior sickle scalers, universal curets have two paired, mirror-image working ends. Both working ends are needed to debride all the tooth surfaces of the mouth. The paired working ends of a universal curet may be found on two single-ended instruments or may be combined on one double-ended instrument. Examples of paired universal curets include: the Columbia 2R/2L; Columbia 13/14; Rule 3/4; Barnhart 1/2; Barnhart 5/6; Younger-Good 7/8; Indiana University 13/14; HU 1/2; Bunting 5/6; Mallery 1/2; Langer 1/2; Langer 3/4; Langer 5/6, and Langer 17/18.

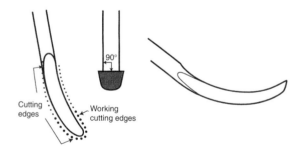

DESIGN CHARACTERISTICS OF UNIVERSAL CURETS

Working end	Curves upward
Cutting edges	Straight; parallel to one another
Relationship of face to shank	Face at 90° angle to lower shank
Number of cutting edges	2 cutting edges per working end
Working end in cross-section	Semi-circular
Functional shank	Designs vary from short to long and rigid to flexible
Application to sextants and surfaces	A single universal curet may be used on all anterior and posterior surfaces
Use on crown and root surfaces	Enamel and cementum surfaces

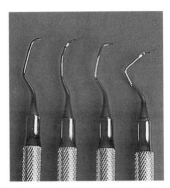

The Langer Universal Curet Series.

The Langer Curet Series was introduced in 1986. The working end of a Langer curet has the design characteristics of a universal curet, a face that is at a 90° angle to the lower shank and two parallel cutting edges.

Langer curets differ from other universal curets in two respects:

1. More than one Langer curet is needed to instrument the entire dentition.
2. These curets have long, complex functional shanks.

A set of four Langer curets is recommended for the dentition because each curet is limited to use in a particular section of the dentition. Langer curets are available in standard, rigid, and styles with slim working ends and extended shanks. Within its area of use, each Langer curet is used like any other universal curet. That is, one working end is used to instrument the facial aspect of a tooth (i.e., D, Fa, M), and the opposite working end is used to instrument the lingual aspect (i.e., D, Li, M) of the same tooth. (Application of a universal curet to the teeth is discussed more fully in Chapter 4 [anterior sextants] and Chapter 5 [posterior curets].)

The Langer 5/6 curet in use on anterior teeth.

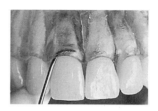

The Langer 1/2 in use on mandibular posterior teeth.

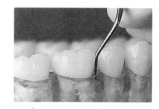

The Langer 3/4 in use on maxillary posterior teeth. (Photos courtesy of Hu-Friedy Manufacturing Company, Inc.)

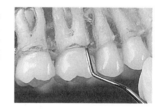

Instrument	Area of Use
Langer 5/6	Mandibular and maxillary anterior teeth
Langer 1/2	Mandibular posterior teeth
Langer 3/4	Maxillary posterior teeth
Langer 17/18	Mandibular and maxillary second and third molars

Area-specific Curets

Area-specific curets are used to remove light subgingival calculus deposits and endotoxins from root surfaces. These instruments have longer functional shanks for access to the middle-third and apical-thirds of the root. The name "area-specific" signifies that each area-specific curet can be applied only to certain surfaces and areas of the mouth.

Area-specific curets have two paired, mirror-image working ends. The paired working ends of an area-specific curet may be found on two single-ended instruments or may be combined on one double-ended instrument. Area-specific curets must be purchased in sets because each instrument is limited to use on specific surfaces or areas of the mouth. Examples of area-specific "sets" include: the Gracey series, Kramer-Nevins series, Turgeon series, Hu-Friedy After Five series, Hu-Friedy Mini Five series, and Hu-Friedy Vision Curvette series.

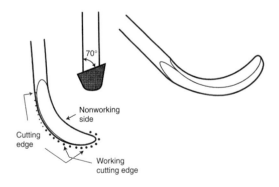

DESIGN CHARACTERISTICS OF AREA-SPECIFIC CURETS

Working end	Curves upward and to one side
Cutting edges	Curved
Relationship of face to shank	Face is tilted in relationship to lower shank
Number of cutting edges	1 cutting edge per working end used on tooth surfaces
Working end in cross-section	Semi-circular
Functional shank	Long or extended shanks in rigid or flexible designs
Application to sextants and surfaces	Single curet is limited to use in certain areas and to certain tooth surfaces
Use on crown and root surfaces	Enamel and cementum surfaces

Designs: Area-specific curets are available in a wide variety of designs. Many designs are modifications based on the standard Gracey curet series, and others are unique design configurations.

Instrument Examples	Design Modification	Design Features
Gracey Finishing curets		Also referred to as "traditional" Gracey curets Original design developed by Dr. Clayton Gracey
Gracey 15/16 curet	Addition to the standard series	Modification of the standard Gracey 11/12 that provides superior access to mesial surfaces of posterior teeth
Gracey Mesial-Distal Curets	New pairing of Gracey curets (double-ended instruments)	This modification changes the way the Gracey 11, 12, 13, and 14 curets are combined on double-ended instruments. The modified combinations, G11/14 and G 12/13, allow the clinician to complete the proximal surfaces on the facial or lingual aspect without changing instruments. For example, the clinician might use the G11/14 to complete the proximal surfaces on the facial aspect of a posterior sextant and the G12/13 for the lingual aspect of the same sextant. **Advantage** = time efficient, no time wasted changing instruments for mesial and distal surfaces.
Gracey Prophy curet series	Modification in shank design	Shank is shorter and more rigid than the Standard series. **Advantage** = will remove medium-sized deposits **Disadvantages** = working end will not reach as far subgingivally because of shorter shank length; less tactile conduction to clinician's fingers because of more rigid shank

Rigid Gracey series	Modification in shank design	Standard series shank length with more rigid shank and working end **Advantage** = will remove medium and tenacious deposits because the rigid shank and working end are less likely to break **Disadvantage** = rigid shank design limits tactile conduction to clinician's hands
Kramer-Nevins series	Modification in working end	Modifications to working end width, curvature, and length **Advantages** = working end provides improved access to difficult areas
DeMarco set Quétin series	Modification in working end	Working ends are reduced to either 0.9 mm or 1.3 mm in width; available in either buccal-lingual or mesial-distal designs **Advantages** = thinner working end provides improved access to proximal root concavities and furcation areas
Hu-Friedy After Five series American Eagle Gracey + 3 Access	Modification in working ends and shanks	Working end is thinner and the lower shank is extended an additional 3 mm in length than standard Gracey series. **Advantages** = slim working end is easier to insert, causes less tissue distention, and provides improved access to root concavities and furcation areas. Extended lower shank allows access to root surface 5 mm or greater apical to the CEJ (cemento-enamel junction). **Disadvantage** = working end might break because of inappropriate use of instrument for medium or large calculus deposits.

continued

Instrument Examples	Design Modification	Design Features
Hu-Friedy Mini Five series American Eagle Gracey + 3 Deep Pocket	Modification in working ends and shanks	Working end is thinner and shortened to half the length of standard Gracey series. The lower shank is extended an additional 3 mm in length than the standard Gracey series. **Advantages** = slim working end is easier to insert; shortened working end provides improved access to root concavities, furcation areas, and midline region on roots of anterior teeth. **Disadvantage** = working end might break because of inappropriate use with medium or large calculus deposits
Turgeon curet series	Modification to working end	Modified working end is thinner and pie-shaped in cross section. **Advantages** = slim working end is easier to insert; modified cross section provides a sharper cutting edge. **Disadvantage** = working end might break because of inappropriate use with medium or large calculus deposits.
Curvette series	Modification to working end and shank	Working end is shorter than the standard Gracey series; the working end has increased curvature. Shank is centered over the round handle, and the lower shank is longer than the standard Gracey series. The shank is marked with bands at 5 and 10 mm. The cutting edge and handles have identification marks. **Advantages** = Shortened working end provides improved access to root concavities and furcation areas. The increased curvature of working end facilitates adaptation to root surfaces; centered working end improves subgingival insertion and increases efficiency of strokes. Bands on shank provide visual guide to depth of working end within pocket. Identification marks allow quick identification of cutting edges and of mesial and distal curets.

The Gracey Curet Series

The first area-specific curet designs were developed in the late 1930's by Dr. Clayton Gracey. These curets represented an important breakthrough in instrument design technology that allowed the clinician to gain access to root surfaces within periodontal pockets without trauma to the pocket epithelium. The Gracey Instrument Series continues to be popular and is the basis for all other area-specific curet designs available today.

Gracey curets are available in standard, prophy, rigid, After Five, and Mini Five styles.

THE GRACEY INSTRUMENT SERIES	
Area of Use	**Gracey Curet**
Anterior sextants	Curet 1 Curet 2 Curet 3 Curet 4
Anterior sextants and premolar teeth	Curet 5 Curet 6
Buccal and lingual surfaces of premolars and molars	Curet 7 Curet 8
Buccal and lingual surfaces of molars	Curet 9 Curet 10
Facial, lingual, and mesial surfaces of posterior teeth	Curet 11 Curet 12
Facial, lingual, and distal surfaces of posterior teeth	Curet 13 Curet 14
Mesial surfaces of posterior teeth	Curet 15 Curet 16
Distal surfaces of posterior teeth	Curet 17 Curet 18

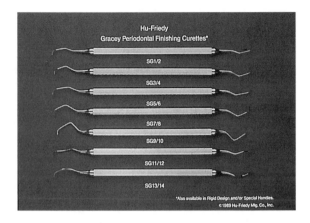

The standard Gracey area-specific curet instrument series. (Photo courtesy of Hu-Friedy Manufacturing Company, Inc.)

Gracey 11/12 and Gracey 15/16

Using a Gracey 11/12, it is sometimes difficult to correctly position the shank parallel to the mesial surface. This is especially true if the patient is unable to open widely. (Photographs of Gracey curets are courtesy of Hu-Friedy Mfg. Co., Inc.)

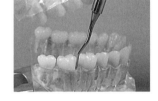

On the Gracey 15/16, the increased angle of the lower shank bend makes it easier to adapt the lower shank to the mesial surface on molar teeth.

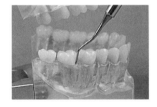

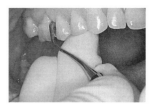

The increased angle of the lower shank bend on the Gracey 15/16 provides superior access in maxillary molar treatment areas.

Gracey 13/14 and Gracey 17/18

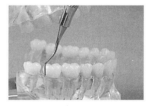

Access to the distal surface of a second molar with a Gracey 13/14 curet can be limited by the patient's inability to open widely. (Photographs of Gracey curets are courtesy of Hu-Friedy Mfg. Co., Inc.)

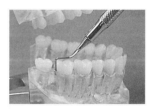

On the Gracey 17/18, the increased angle of the lower shank bend improves access to the distal surfaces of molars.

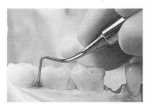

The Gracey 17/18 on a skull. Access to distal surfaces is improved through the multiple exaggerated shank bends of the instrument.

Area-Specific Curets with Modified Design of the Shank and Working End

Recently the design features of the standard area–specific curet have been altered to allow increased access to the middle-third and apical-third of the root surface. The new styles resulted from changes in the design characteristics of the working end and the shank.

1. **Area-specific curets with thinner working ends and longer lower shanks.** The thinner working ends of these instruments are easier to insert under the gingival margin when the tissue is closely adapted to the tooth surface. The lower shank has been extended several millimeters in length to facilitate access to the base of deep periodontal pockets. Examples of this style include the Hu-Friedy After Five Gracey curets and the American Eagle Gracey +3 Access Curettes.

2. **Area-specific curets with shorter, thinner working ends and longer lower shanks.** In addition to being thinner, the working end of these instruments is shortened to half the length of a standard area-specific curet. This thinner, shorter working end is easier to use in deep, narrow pockets and furcation areas. Examples of this style include the Hu-Friedy Mini Five Gracey curets and the American Eagle Gracey +3 Deep Pocket Curettes.

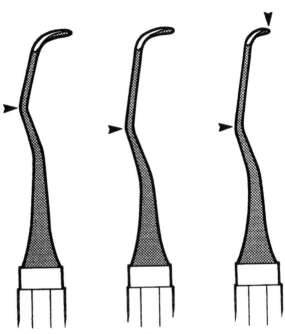

Area-specific curet

Area-specific curet with a thinner working end and an extended lower shank

Area-specific curet with a shorter, thinner tip and an extended lower shank

Curvette Area-Specific Curets

The design characteristics of curvette curets differ from those of standard Gracey curets in several respects: (1) 50% shorter working end, (2) increased curvature of the working end, (3) straighter shank on anterior instruments, and (4) extended lower shank on posterior instruments.

The shorter working end of the curvette curet provides improved access to root concavities, furcation areas of posterior teeth, and midlines of anterior teeth. The increased curvature of the working end facilitates adaptation to curved root surfaces. Ergonomic features of the curvette series are markings on the shank and working end identification marks. A raised band on the shank at 5 and 10 mm helps the clinician visually assess pocket depth during instrumentation. A small "X" on the handle visually indicates the lower cutting edge; this feature assists the clinician in quick identification of these smaller working ends.

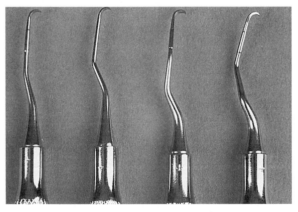

The Curvette series of area-specific curets.

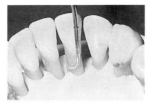

Use of a Vision Curvette Sub-Zero on anterior teeth. (Courtesy of Hu-Friedy Manufacturing Co., Inc.)

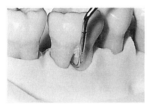

Use of a Vision Curvette 13/14 in a furcation area of a posterior tooth. Band markings on the shank at 5 and 10 mm provide a visual indication of the depth of the working end within a periodontal pocket. (Courtesy of Hu-Friedy Manufacturing Co., Inc.)

Instrument	Area of Use
Curvette Sub-Zero	Anterior teeth and premolars
Curvette 1/2	Anterior teeth and premolars
Curvette 11/12	Mesial surfaces of molars
Curvette 13/14	Distal surfaces of molars

Section 4:

Analysis of Instrument Design Features

SICKLE SCALERS

Design Features: Sickle Scaler	Analysis of Design Feature
Working end has flat face with no upward curvature	**Advantage** = none **Disadvantage** = does not adapt to convex or concave tooth surfaces
Lateral surfaces meet in a pointed tip	**Advantage** = pointed tip provides good access to the supragingival proximal surfaces, especially on mandibular anteriors. **Disadvantage** = leading third of the cutting edge does not adapt well to curved tooth surfaces; sharp point can gouge cemental surfaces, and use is not recommended on cemental surfaces.
Face is perpendicular to the lower shank	**Advantage** = efficient; two cutting edges per working end can be used for calculus removal **Disadvantage** = level cutting edges are not self-angulated to contact the tooth at a 70° to 80° angle; should not be used subgingivally
Pointed back and tip	**Advantage** = none **Disadvantage** = should not be used subgingivally

continued

Design Features: Sickle Scaler	Analysis of Design Feature
Short shank length	**Advantage** = shank is strong for removal of large calculus deposits. **Disadvantage** = limited to use on crowns of teeth
Rigid shank	**Advantage** = strong shank for removal of large calculus deposits; strong shank will not bend or "spring" with firm pressure during a calculus removal stroke **Disadvantage** = provides limited tactile information to the clinician's fingers

UNIVERSAL CURETS

Design Features: Universal Curet	Analysis of Design Feature
Working end has an upward curvature	**Advantage** = curved face adapts to convex tooth surfaces for easy insertion beneath the gingival margin. **Disadvantage** = none
Lateral surfaces are straight	**Advantage** = none **Disadvantage** = leading third of cutting edge is straight and, therefore, doesn't adapt well to concave and convex root surfaces.

continued

Design Features: Universal Curet	Analysis of Design Feature
Lateral surfaces meet in a rounded toe	**Advantage** = much less likely to gouge cemental surfaces; adapts better to root curvatures than the pointed toe of the sickle scaler **Disadvantage** = rounded tip is wider than a pointed tip and, therefore, is more difficult to adapt to the proximal surfaces of overlapping or closely adapted adjacent teeth.
Face is perpendicular to the lower shank	**Advantage** = efficient two cutting edges per working end can be used for calculus removal. **Disadvantage** = level cutting edges are not self-angulated; more difficult to use in pocket when tissue is closely adapted to tooth than is an area-specific curet
Rounded back	**Advantage** = can be inserted beneath the gingival margin without tissue trauma **Disadvantage** = none
Medium or long shank length	**Advantage** = provides access to the cervical-third of the root **Disadvantage** = less effective in accessing the middle-third of the root
Rigid or medium shank	**Advantage** = shank is strong for removal of medium calculus deposits. **Disadvantage** = provides fair tactile information to clinician's fingers

AREA-SPECIFIC CURETS

Design Features: Area-Specific Curet	Analysis of Design Feature
Working end has an upward curvature	**Advantage** = curved face adapts to convex tooth surfaces for easy insertion beneath the gingival margin. **Disadvantage** = none
Lateral surfaces are curved	**Advantage** = curved cutting edge provides improved adaptation to concave and convex root surfaces. **Disadvantage** = none
Lateral surfaces meet in a rounded toe	**Advantage** = much less likely to gouge cemental surfaces; adapts better to root curvatures than the pointed toe of the sickle scaler **Disadvantage** = rounded tip is wider than a pointed tip and, therefore, is more difficult to adapt to the proximal surfaces of closely adapted adjacent teeth
Face is offset in relation to the lower shank	**Advantage** = cutting edge is self-angulated; readily used subgingivally without tissue trauma **Disadvantage** = only one cutting edge per working end can be used for root surface debridement; less time efficient
Rounded back	**Advantage** = can be inserted beneath the gingival margin without tissue trauma **Disadvantage** = none

continued

Design Features: Area-Specific Curet	Analysis of Design Feature
Long, complex shank	**Advantage** = provides best access to root surfaces of any hand-activated debridement instrument **Disadvantage** = none
Flexible shank design	**Advantage** = provides good tactile information to the clinician's fingers **Disadvantage** = instruments with flexible shanks should be limited to use for removal of light calculus and endotoxins. [Note: most area-specific designs also are available in modified designs with rigid shanks.]

Section 5:

References and Suggested Readings

<u>Also refer to References and Suggested Readings for
Chapters 4, 5, and 6.</u>

Anderson, G.B., Palmer, J.A., Bye, F.L., Smith, B.A., Caffesse, R.G.: Effectiveness of subgingival scaling and root planing: single versus multiple episodes of instrumentation. J Periodontol Apr;67(4):367-73, 1996.

Balevi, B.: Engineering specifics of the periodontal curet's cutting edge. J Periodontol Apr;67(4):374-8, 1996.

Burkhart, N.W., Crawford, J.: Critical steps in instrument cleaning: removing debris after sonication. J Am Dent Assoc Apr;128(4):456-63, 1997.

Cheetham, W.A., Wilson, M., Kieser, J.B.: Root surface debridement—an in vitro assessment. J Clin Periodontol May;15(5):288-92, 1988.

Cobb, C.M.: Non-surgical pocket therapy: mechanical. Ann Periodontol Nov;1(1):443-90, 1996.

Cross-Poline, G.N., Stach, D.J., Newman, S.M.: Effects of curet and ultrasonics on root surfaces. Am J Dent Jun;8(3):131-3, 1995.

Dragoo, M.R., Wheeler, B.G.: Clinical evaluation of subgingival debridement with ultrasonic instruments used by trained and untrained operators. Gen Dent May-Jun;44(3):234-7, 1996.

Ebersole, J.L., Cappelli, D., Steffen, M.J., Willmann, D.E., O'Dell, D.S.: Host response assessment in recurring periodontitis. J Clin Periodontol Mar;23(3 Pt 2):258-62, 1996.

Ebersole, J.L., Taubman, M.A., Smith, D.J., Haffajee, A.D.: Effect of subgingival scaling on systemic antibody responses to oral microorganisms. Infect Immun May;48(2):534-9, 1985.

Efeoglu, E., Sandalli, P.: A 14-year follow-up study of localized juvenile periodontitis treated by scaling and root planing, systemic metronidazole, and subgingival curettage: a case report. Periodontol Clin Invest Fall;18(2):6-12, 1996.

Fujikawa, K., O'Leary, T.J., Kafrawy, A.H.: The effect of retained subgingival calculus on healing after flap surgery. J Periodontol Mar;59(3):170-5, 1988.

Gantes, B.G., Nilveus, R., Lie, T., Leknes, K.N.: The effect of hygiene instruments on dentin surfaces: scanning electron microscopic observations. J Periodontol Mar;63(3):151-7, 1992.

Gmur, R., Saxer, U.P., Guggenheim, B.: Effects of blunt scaling on periodontal status and subgingival microorganisms. A pilot study. Schweiz Monatsschr Zahnmed 104(4):430-9, 1994.

Greenstein, G.: Periodontal response to mechanical non-surgical therapy: a review. J Periodontol Feb;63(2):118-30, 1992.

Haffajee, A.D., Cugini, M.A., Dibart, S., Smith, C., Kent, R.L. Jr., Socransky, S.S.: The effect of SRP (scaling and root planing) on the clinical and microbiological parameters of periodontal diseases. J Clin Periodontol May;24(5):324-34, 1997.

Hughes, F.J., Auger, D.W., Smales, F.C.: Investigation of the distribution of cementum-associated lipopolysaccharides in periodontal disease by scanning electron microscope immunohistochemistry. J Periodontal Res Mar;23(2):100-6, 1988.

Jeffcoat, M.K., McGuire, M., Newman, M.G.: Evidence-based periodontal treatment. Highlights from the 1996 World Workshop in Periodontics. J Am Dent Assoc Jun;128(6):713-24, 1997.

Kepic, T.J., O'Leary, T.J., Kafrawy, A.H.: Total calculus removal: an attainable objective? J Periodontol Jan;61(1):16-20, 1990.

Kinane, D.F., Radvar, M.: The effect of smoking on mechanical and antimicrobial periodontal therapy. J Periodontol May;68(5):467-72, 1997.

Leknes, KN.: The influence of anatomic and iatrogenic root surface characteristics on bacterial colonization and periodontal destruction: A review. J Periodontol Jun;68(6):507-16, 1997.

Leknes, K.N., Lie, T., Wikesjo, U.M., Boe, O.E., Selvig, K.A.: Influence of tooth instrumentation roughness on subgingival microbial colonization. J Periodontol Apr;65(4):303-8, 1994.

Nakib, N.M., Bissada, N.F., Simmelink, J.W., Goldstine, S.N.: Endotoxin penetration into root cementum of periodontally healthy and diseased human teeth. J Periodontol Jun;53(6):368-78, 1982.

Oberholzer, R., Rateitschak, K.H.: Root cleaning or root smoothing: An in vivo study. J Clin Periodontol Jun;23(4):326-30, 1996.

O'Hehir, T.E.: Basic science is changing the way we practice dental hygiene. RDH Jan;15(1):11, 1995.

O'Hehir, TE: Periodontal debridement therapy. Access, Am Dent Hygienists' Assoc May-June;9:49, 1995.

O'Hehir, T.E.: Curettes not effective in debridement of furcations. RDH Jun;14(6):32, 1994.

O'Hehir, T.E.: Overhang removal should be integral part of debridement. RDH Jan;14(1):38, 1994.

O'Hehir, T.E.: Studies show similar results with surgical and non-surgical therapy. RDH Sep;13(9):42, 44, 1993.

O'Hehir, T.E.: Calculus removal should be based on body's reaction, not thoroughness. RDH Mar;13(3):23, 1993.

O'Hehir, T.E.: Studies question extensive root planing to remove cementum. RDH Jul;12(7):46, 1992.

O'Leary, R., Sved, A.M., Davies, E.H., Leighton, T.G., Wilson, M., Kieser, J.B.: The bactericidal effects of dental ultrasound on Actinobacillus actinomycetemcomitans and Porphyromonas gingivalis: An in vitro investigation. J Clin Periodontol Jun;24(6):432-9, 1997.

Pasquini, R., Clark, S.M., Baradaran, S., Adams, D.F.: Periodontal files—a comparative study. J Periodontol Dec;66(12):1040-6, 1995.

Proceedings of the 1996 World Workshop in Periodontics. Lansdowne, VA: July 13-17, 1996. Ann Periodontol Nov;1(1):1-947, 1996.

Shiloah, J., Patters, M.R.: DNA probe analyses of the survival of selected periodontal pathogens following scaling, root planing, and intrapocket irrigation. J Periodontol Jun;65(6):568-75, 1994.

White, D.J., Cox, E.R., Arends, J., Nieborg, J.H., Leydsman, H., Wieringa, D.W., Dijkman, A.G., Ruben, J.R.: Instruments and methods for the quantitative measurement of factors affecting hygienist/dentist efforts during scaling and root planing of the teeth. J Clin Dent;7(2 Spec No):32-40, 1996.

Yukna, R.A., Scott, J.B., Aichelmann-Reidy, M.E., LeBlanc, D.M., Mayer, E.T.: Clinical evaluation of the speed and effectiveness of subgingival calculus removal on single-rooted teeth with diamond-coated ultrasonic tips. J Periodontol May;68(5):436-42, 1997.

4

Periodontal Debridement in Anterior Sextants

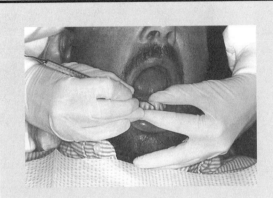

In this chapter

Section 1:

Sequence for Instrumentation

ANTERIOR SEXTANTS, RIGHT-HANDED CLINICIAN

Anterior Sextants

Facial Aspect, Surfaces Toward

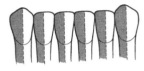

Mentally divide the facial aspect into surfaces toward you and away from you. On this illustration, the shaded surfaces are the surfaces toward you. The surfaces toward you will be done first.

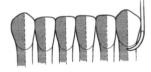

Begin with the mandibular left canine. Place the leading-third of the cutting edge at the midline of the tooth. Make strokes across the facial and proximal surface. End with strokes under the contact area of the mesial surface.

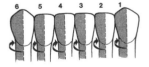

Complete the **facial surfaces toward you** in the following sequence:

1. Left canine
2. Left lateral incisor
3. Left central incisor
4. Right central incisor
5. Right lateral incisor
6. Right canine

Facial Aspect, Surfaces Away

Complete **the facial surfaces away** in the following sequence:

7. Right canine
8. Right lateral incisor
9. Right central incisor
10. Left central incisor
11. Left lateral incisor
12. Left canine

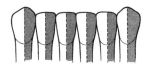

Lingual Aspect, Surfaces Toward

The lingual aspect is completed in a similar manner to the facial aspect. Complete the surfaces toward you and then the surfaces away from you.

ANTERIOR SEXTANTS, LEFT-HANDED CLINICIAN

Mandibular Anteriors

Facial Aspect, Surfaces Toward

Mentally divide the facial aspect into surfaces toward you and away from you. On this illustration, the shaded surfaces are the surfaces toward you. The surfaces toward you will be done first.

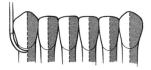

Begin with the mandibular right canine. Place the leading-third of the cutting edge at the midline of the tooth. Make strokes across the facial and on to the proximal surface. End with strokes under the contact area of the mesial surface.

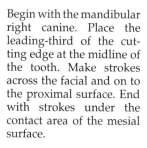

Complete the **facial surfaces toward you** in the following sequence:

1. Right canine
2. Right lateral incisor
3. Right central incisor
4. Left central incisor
5. Left lateral incisor
6. Left canine

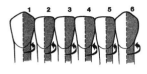

Facial Aspect, Surfaces Away

Complete **the facial surfaces away** in the following sequence:

7. Left canine
8. Left lateral incisor
9. Left central incisor
10. Right central incisor
11. Right lateral incisor
12. Right canine

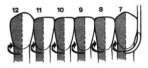

Lingual Aspect, Surfaces Toward

The lingual aspect is completed in a similar manner to the facial aspect. Complete the surfaces toward you and then the surfaces away from you.

Section 2:

Use of Universal Curets

CUTTING EDGES: UNIVERSAL CURETS

Universal curets may be used on enamel and cemental surfaces. One double-ended universal curet can be used to instrument all surfaces of an anterior sextant.

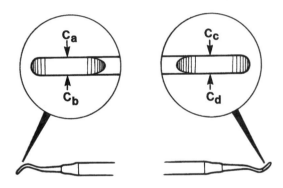

Cutting Edges

A universal curet has two paired working ends. Each working end has 2 cutting edges: C_a and C_b or C_c and C_d.

Facial

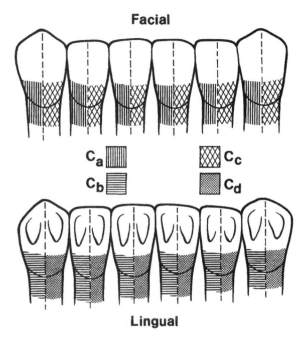

Lingual

Universal Curet: Application of Cutting Edges to Anterior Tooth Surfaces

All four cutting edges are required to debride the anterior surfaces (maxillary and mandibular facial and lingual aspects).

For example, if cutting edge C_a is used on the *facial aspect, surfaces **toward** you,* then:

- Cutting edge C_c is used on the *facial aspect, surfaces **away**,*
- Cutting edge C_b is used on the *lingual aspect, surfaces **toward** you,* and
- Cutting edge C_d is used on the *lingual aspect, surfaces **away**.*

SELECTING THE CORRECT CUTTING EDGE OF A UNIVERSAL CURET

When using a universal curet, you must identify which of the four cutting edges is the correct one for use on a particular surface. Use these steps to select the correct cutting edge.

STEPS FOR SELECTING THE CORRECT CUTTING EDGE OF A UNIVERSAL CURET ON ANTERIOR TOOTH SURFACES

1. Grasp the instrument in a modified pen grasp, and establish a fulcrum.

2. Place either working end on the tooth surface on which you wish to work.

3. Hold the instrument so that the **handle is parallel to the long axis** of the tooth surface on which you wish to work.

4. Look closely at the working end that is adapted against the tooth surface.

   If the instrument **face tilts away from** the tooth surface, this is the **incorrect cutting edge** for this tooth surface. Both cutting edges on this working end are incorrect for use on this tooth surface.

   If the instrument **face tilts toward** the tooth, this is the **correct cutting edge** for this tooth surface.

   RULE: For anterior teeth the *face* of the working end should tilt *toward* the tooth.

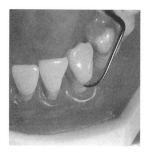 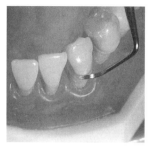

Correct: Face tilted toward surface on which you plan to work when handle is parallel to tooth surface.

Incorrect: Face tilted away from surface on which you plan to work when handle is parallel to tooth surface.

USE OF UNIVERSAL CURET ON ANTERIOR TOOTH SURFACES

Example: Mandibular Anteriors, Facial Aspect

Beginning on page 206, the step-by-step approach to using a universal curet on anterior teeth is shown for the facial aspect of the mandibular left anteriors, mesial surfaces, and the mandibular right anteriors, distal surfaces. Debridement of the remaining surfaces of the mandibular anteriors and the maxillary anteriors is done in a similar manner.

Select the correct cutting edge for use on the facial aspect of the mandibular left canine, working from the midline of the facial and on to the mesial surface.

Establish a 70° to 80° instrument face-to-tooth surface angulation, and engage the cutting edge against the tooth.

Push down with your fulcrum finger and activate a working stroke.

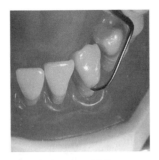

Relax your grasp. Roll the instrument handle to adapt the working end to the next section of the tooth.

Establish correct angulation, and activate a stroke.

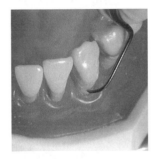

Roll the instrument handle to obtain proper adaptation to the mesio-facial line angle.

Establish correct angulation, and activate a stroke.

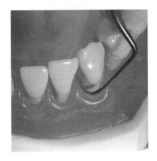

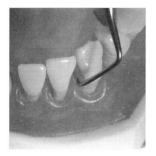

Relax your grasp, and roll the instrument handle to adapt to the mesial surface.

Angulate, engage the cutting edge, and activate a stroke.

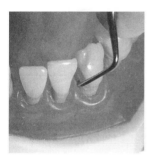

Continue strokes until the facial half of the mesial proximal surface has been covered.

Section 3:

Use of Area-Specific Curets

Area-specific curets may be used on enamel and cemental surfaces. One double-ended area-specific curet is needed to instrument all surfaces of an anterior sextant.

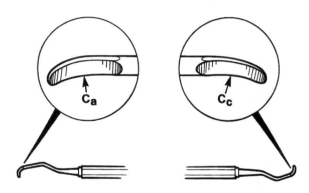

Cutting Edges

An area-specific curet has two paired working ends. Only one cutting edge on each working end (i.e., C_a or C_c) is used for tooth surface debridement.

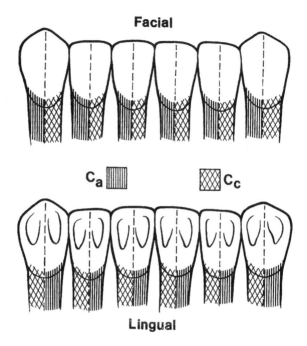

Application of Cutting Edges to Anterior Tooth Surfaces

For example, if cutting edge C_a is used on the *facial aspect, surfaces **toward** you,* then:

- Cutting edge C_c is used on the *facial aspect, surfaces **away**,*
- Cutting edge C_c is used on the *lingual aspect, surfaces **toward** you,* and
- Cutting edge C_a is used on the *lingual aspect, surfaces **away**.*

SELECTING THE CORRECT CUTTING EDGE OF AN AREA-SPECIFIC CURET

STEPS FOR SELECTING THE CORRECT CUTTING EDGE OF AN AREA-SPECIFIC CURET ON ANTERIOR TOOTH SURFACES

1. Grasp the instrument in a modified pen grasp, and establish a fulcrum.

2. Place either working end on the tooth surface on which you wish to work.

3. Hold the instrument so that the **lower shank is parallel to the tooth surface** on which you wish to work.

4. Look closely at the working end that is adapted against the tooth surface.

   If the instrument **face tilts away from** the tooth surface, this is the **incorrect cutting edge** for this tooth surface. Both cutting edges on this working end are incorrect for use on this tooth surface.

   If the instrument **face tilts toward** the tooth, this is the **correct cutting edge** for this tooth surface.

   RULE: For anterior teeth the *face* of the working end should tilt *toward* the tooth.

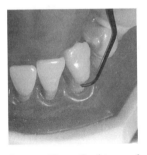

Correct: Face tilted toward surface on which you plan to work when the lower shank is parallel to the tooth surface.

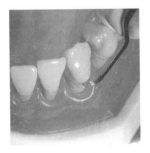

Incorrect: Face tilted away from surface on which you plan to work when the lower shank is parallel to the tooth surface.

Identifying the Cutting Edge for
Tooth-Surface Debridement

Only one cutting edge per working end of an area-specific curet is used to debride the coronal and root surfaces of teeth. To identify this cutting edge, hold an area-specific curet so you are looking at the toe of the working end. Raise or lower the instrument handle until the shank nearest the working end is perpendicular to the floor. With the working end in this position, one cutting edge is tilted toward the terminal shank; the other, tilts away from the terminal shank. *The cutting edge that tilts away from the terminal shank is the one designed for tooth-surface debridement.* Other ways of describing this cutting edge include: the lower cutting edge, the outside cutting edge, and the longer cutting edge.

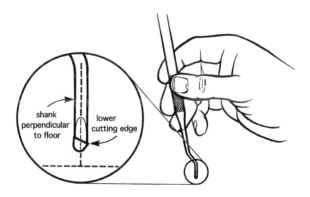

USE OF AN AREA-SPECIFIC CURET ON ANTERIOR TOOTH SURFACES

The step-by-step approach to using an area-specific curet on anterior teeth is shown for the facial aspect of the mandibular left anteriors, mesial surfaces, and the mandibular right anteriors, distal surfaces. Debridement of the remaining surfaces of the mandibular anteriors and the maxillary anteriors is done in a similar manner.

Select the correct cutting edge for use on the facial aspect of the mandibular left canine, working from the midline of the facial and on to the mesial surface.

Establish a 70° to 80° instrument face-to-tooth surface angulation, and engage the cutting edge against the tooth.

Push down with your fulcrum finger, and activate a working stroke.

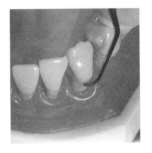

Relax your grasp. Roll the instrument handle to adapt the working end to the next area.

Establish correct angulation, and activate a stroke.

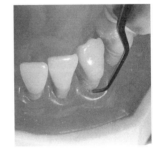

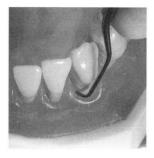

Roll the instrument handle to obtain proper adaptation to the mesio-facial line angle.

Establish correct angulation, and activate a stroke.

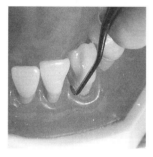

Relax your grasp, and roll the instrument handle to adapt to the mesial surface.

Angulate, engage the cutting edge, and activate a stroke.

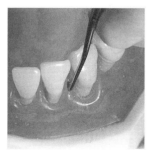

Continue strokes until the facial half of the mesial proximal surface has been covered.

Section 4:

Root Surface Debridement

MULTIDIRECTIONAL WORK STROKES

Light multidirectional work strokes are used to remove residual calculus granules and bacterial byproducts from the surface of the cementum. Multidirectional strokes are achieved by employing all three stroke directions, one-by-one in succession.

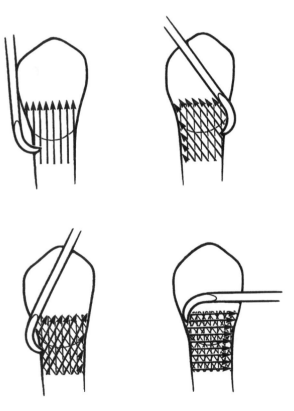

ROOT SURFACE DEBRIDEMENT OF ANTERIOR TEETH

It is important to have a defined knowledge of root morphology in order to debride the root surfaces effectively. The majority of instrumentation is done on root surfaces that are hidden from view within a pathologically deepened sulcus (i.e., periodontal pocket). A clear mental picture of root anatomy and a keen tactile sense are necessary for periodontal instrumentation to be successful.

A root concavity is a linear developmental depression in the root surface. Root concavities commonly occur on the proximal surfaces of anterior teeth.

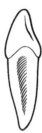

A long depression extends along the mesial root surface of this mandibular canine.

This concavity begins near the CEJ (cemento-enamel junction) and extends along the entire length of the mesial root surface.

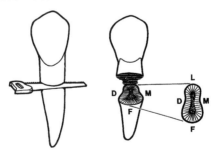

In cross section, the root of this canine is seen to have two root concavities: one concavity on the mesial root surface and one on the distal root surface.

INSTRUMENTATION OF ROOT CONCAVITIES

A piece of floss stretched around a root surface will not disrupt bacterial plaque in a proximal root concavity.

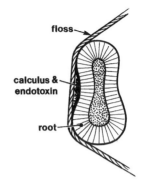

The same problem occurs when the clinician does not consider root morphology during instrumentation. The length of the cutting edge spans the depression leaving calculus deposits undisturbed.

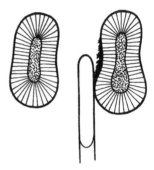

The clinician should roll the instrument handle to direct the leading-third of the cutting edge into the depression.

Notice that the middle- and heel-thirds of the cutting edge are rotated toward the adjacent tooth.

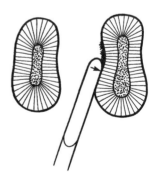

ROOT MORPHOLOGY REVIEW: ANTERIOR TEETH

Mandibular Central Incisor

Mesial surface of root = shallow depression sometimes present in cervical area; deep linear concavity extending the length of root

Mandibular Central Incisor

Distal surface of root = shallow depression sometimes present in cervical area; deep linear concavity extending the length of root

Mandibular Lateral Incisor

Mesial surface of root = shallow depression sometimes present in cervical area; linear concavity extending the length of root

Mandibular Lateral Incisor

Distal surface of root = shallow depression sometimes present in cervical area; linear concavity extending the length of root

Mandibular Canine

Mesial surface of root = no depression in cervical area; deep linear concavity extending the length of root

Mandibular Canine

Distal surface of root = no depression in cervical area; deep linear concavity extending the length of root

Maxillary Central Incisor

Mesial surface of the root = cervical area of root is smooth; usually no root concavity

Maxillary Central Incisor

Distal surface of the root = cervical area of root is smooth; usually no root concavity

Maxillary Lateral Incisor

Mesial and distal surfaces of the root = shallow depression sometimes present in cervical area of root; linear concavity usually present

Maxillary Lateral Incisor

Cervical area of lingual surface = if palatal groove is present on cingulum of crown, it may extend onto the cervical third of the lingual root surface

Maxillary Canine

Mesial surface of the root = depression in cervical-third; deep linear concavity extending the length of the root

Maxillary Canine

Distal surface of the root = depression in cervical-third; deep linear concavity extending the length of the root

Section 5:

Problem Identification–Difficulties in Instrumentation of Anterior Teeth

Problem	Causes Listed in order from most to least likely cause for each problem
A. Difficulty obtaining vision of the anterior teeth	1. Positioning: patient chair is too high in relationship to the seated clinician, which is causing the clinician to raise shoulders and arms to reach treatment area and strain in order to see the area. 2. Positioning: patient's head is not in the correct position for the treatment area (i.e., chin up or down, turned toward or away). 3. Positioning: top of patient's head is not even with the top edge of headrest, which is causing the clinician to stretch (when seated directly behind the patient) in order to reach treatment area for surfaces away from the clinician. 4. Positioning: clinician is not in appropriate operator position for surfaces (i.e., toward or away).
B. Difficulty obtaining vision of the lingual aspect of anterior teeth	1. Positioning: patient's head is not in a chin-down position. 2. Mirror: mirror is not used, positioned too close to the lingual surfaces of teeth, or not rotated to allow vision of proximal surfaces. 3. All of the causes listed under **Problem A.**

continued

Problem	Causes Listed in order from most to least likely cause for each problem
C. Difficulty gaining access to a tooth surface with the instrument working end	1. Most likely causes listed under **Problem A.** 2. Likely causes listed under **Problem B.** 3. Retraction: if working on facial aspect, retraction of lips is not adequate. 4. Fulcrum: finger rest is too close to area being instrumented so that the finger blocks view. 5. Clinician's hand: hand is blocking view (i.e., could be mirror hand or instrument hand). 6. Grasp: clinician has incorrect technique with grasp.
D. Calculus deposits missed on proximal surfaces	1. Mirror: mirror is not rotated to view the proximal surfaces from various angles; this is especially common for the lingual aspect of the mandibular anteriors. 2. Clinician is not using any basic skill, i.e., position, grasp, fulcrum, activation, and adaptation. 3. Design: clinician is not selecting an appropriate instrument for the location or type of calculus. 4. Working end: clinician is not selecting the correct working end and cutting edge for surface. 5. Adaptation: clinician is not rolling instrument handle to adapt the leading-third of the cutting edge against the proximal surface. 6. Adaptation in root concavity: clinician is not rolling instrument handle to direct the leading-third of the cutting edge into the root concavity. 7. Adaptation on proximal surface: clinician is not extending the working strokes at least halfway across the proximal surface from the facial and lingual aspects of tooth.

continued

Problem	Causes Listed in order from most to least likely cause for each problem
E. Calculus deposits missed at midline region of anterior tooth	1. Stroke: clinician is not overlapping working strokes. 2. Stroke direction: clinician is not using a circumferential (i.e., horizontal) stroke at the midline on the facial or lingual aspect with a curet.
F. Interdental papillae lacerated	1. Handle roll: clinician is not rolling handle to reestablish adaptation of the leading-third of the cutting edge when making strokes in the line angle region of the tooth. 2. Adaptation: clinician is attempting to adapt too much of the length of the cutting edge to the tooth, especially in the region of the line angle.
G. Lack of strength or control with work stroke	1. Grasp: instrument handle is supported only by the pads of the index finger and thumb in "pinching" type of grasp; midsection of the handle is not resting against the side of the index finger for support. 2. Grasp: fingers are spread apart, the fulcrum finger is not in contact with other fingers, and the hand is not functioning as a unit. 3. Fulcrum finger: ring finger does not maintain pressure against the rest point on the tooth throughout the stroke; ring finger may actually lift away from the tooth. 4. Fulcrum finger: ring finger is limp and does not act as the "support beam for the hand" during the stroke.

continued

Problem	Causes Listed in order from most to least likely cause for each problem
	5. Fulcrum: rest point is too far away or too close to the tooth being instrumented for the size of this clinician's hands and the length of the fingers. 6. Finger rest: rest is not stable and may be on gingiva or on the facial or lingual surface rather than on the incisal surface, labio-, or linguo-incisal line angle of the tooth. 7. Position: clinician has arm pressed against his or her torso so that the arm or wrist motion is restricted. 8. Activation: when making a calculus removal stroke, the clinician fails to apply pressure against the handle with the index finger (or thumb) to engage cutting edge on tooth. 9. Activation: work strokes are too long causing loss of control. 10. Activation: force of stroke is not in coronal direction or not limited to a coronal direction (force may be in a push and pull direction). 11. Activation: clinician is working too rapidly and making strokes too quickly.
H. Poor tactile discrimination	1. Grasp: middle finger is pressing against shank rather than resting lightly on the shank. 2. Grasp: clinician is holding the handle too tightly (i.e., "death grip").

continued

Problem	Causes Listed in order from most to least likely cause for each problem
	3. Grasp: index finger and thumb are not opposite each other on the handle. A common problem is holding the index finger on the midsection of handle, whereas the thumb and middle finger are actually being used to hold the instrument. This grasp makes it difficult to roll the handle and also greatly diminishes tactile sensitivity because the middle finger is not resting on the shank.
	4. Assessment stroke: clinician is not using feather-light, overlapping strokes that cover every square millimeter of the tooth surface.
	5. Assessment stroke: clinician is not beginning stroke at the base of sulcus or pocket (i.e., working end not inserted to base).
	6. Handle roll: clinician is not reestablishing adaptation of the leading-third of working end in the line angle region of tooth by rolling the handle.
	7. Stroke: clinician is not extending strokes at least halfway across the proximal surface area from the facial and lingual aspects of the tooth.
I. Inability to obtain adaptation of cutting edge to surface	1. Most common cause is inability to gain access to area; refer to **Problem C.**
	2. Common problem is inability to obtain vision of the treatment area; refer to **Problem A.**
	3. Adaptation: clinician is attempting to adapt too much of the length of the cutting edge.
	4. Instrument design: clinician is not selecting an appropriate instrument for the task.

continued

Problem	Causes Listed in order from most to least likely cause for each problem
	5. Also refer to **Problem J,** difficulties in adaptation.
J. Difficulties in maintaining adaptation	1. Refer to **Problem I** if the problem is in attaining adaptation. 2. Grasp: imprecise grasp makes it difficult for the clinician to maintain adaptation, especially when the: a) index finger and thumb are not opposite each other on the handle. A common problem is holding the index finger on the midsection of the handle, whereas the thumb and middle finger are actually being used to hold the instrument. This grasp makes it difficult to roll the handle, and it also greatly diminishes tactile sensitivity. b) clinician fails to reposition fingers slightly on the handle after rolling it, thus fingers become "tangled up" or "wrapped around each other." 3. Parallelism in mesial-distal plane: clinician cannot keep handle parallel by adjusting hand position. As the clinician moves from tooth to tooth across an anterior sextant (working closer and closer to himself or herself), she or he fails to reposition the hand and fulcrum closer to the surface being instrumented. 4. Parallelism in labial-lingual plane: clinician cannot keep handle as parallel as possible to the long axis of tooth causing the face, rather than cutting edge, to be in contact with the tooth.

Section 6:

References and Suggested Readings

Also refer to References and Suggested Readings for Chapters 3 and 6.

Aoki, A., Ando, Y., Watanabe, H., Ishikawa, I.: In vitro studies on laser scaling of subgingival calculus with an erbium: YAG laser. J Periodontol Dec;65(12):1097-106, 1994.

Ash, M.: Wheeler's dental anatomy, physiology and occlusion. Philadelphia, PA: W.B. Saunders, 1993.

Blank, L.W., Rule, J.T., Colangelo, G.A., Copelan, N.S., Perlich, M.A.: The relationship between first presentation and subsequent observations in heavy calculus formers. J Periodontol 1994 Aug;65(8): 750-4.

Brand, R., Isselhard, D.: Anatomy of orofacial structures. St. Louis, MO: C.V. Mosby Co., 1990.

Canis, M.F., Kramer, G.M., Pameijer, C.M.: Calculus attachment. Review of the literature and new findings. J Periodontol Aug;50(8):406-15, 1979.

Gher, M.W. Jr., Vernino, A.R.: Root anatomy: a local factor in inflammatory periodontal disease. Int J Periodontics Restorative Dent;1(5):52-63, 1981.

Gher, M.W. Jr., Vernino, A.R.: Root morphology—clinical significance in pathogenesis and treatment of periodontal disease. J Am Dent Assoc Oct;101(4):627-33, 1980.

Hou, G.L., Tsai, C.C.: Clinical significance of tooth morphology correlated with periodontal disease—I. Kao Hsiung I Hsueh Ko Hsueh Tsa Chih Apr;13(4):200-12, 1997.

Macpherson, L.M., Girardin, D.C., Hughes, N.J., Stephen, K.W., Dawes, C.: The site-specificity of supragingival calculus deposition on the lingual surfaces of the six permanent lower anterior teeth in humans and the effects of age, sex, gum-chewing habits, and the time since the last prophylaxis on calculus scores. J Dent Res Oct;74(10):1715-20, 1995.

Mandel, I.D.: Calculus update: prevalence, pathogenicity and prevention. J Am Dent Assoc May;126(5):573-80, 1995.

Marklund, M., Persson, M.: The relationship between mandibular morphology and apical root curvature in man. Arch Oral Biol;33(6):391-4, 1988.

McKechnie, L. B.: Root morphology in periodontal therapy. Dent Hygienist News;6,(1):3-6, 1993.

Nancollas, G.H., Johnsson, M.A.: Calculus formation and inhibition. Adv Dent Res Jul;8(2):307-11, 1994.

Woefel, J.: Dental anatomy: Its relevance to dentistry, 4th ed. Philadelphia, PA: Lea & Febiger, 1990.

5

Periodontal Debridement in Posterior Sextants

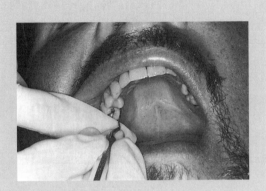

In this chapter

Section 1:

Use of Universal Curets

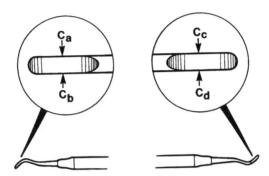

Cutting Edges: A posterior universal curet has two paired working ends. Each working end has 2 cutting edges, C_a and C_b or C_c and C_d.

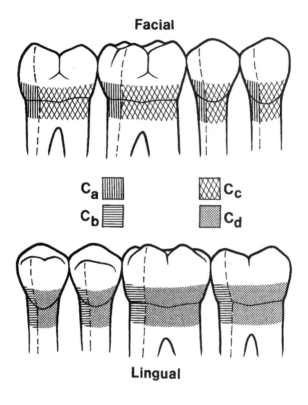

Facial

C_a | | | | |
C_b ▭
▨ C_c
▦ C_d

Lingual

APPLICATION OF A UNIVERSAL CURET TO POSTERIOR TOOTH SURFACES

The two cutting edges, C_a and C_b, of working end A are used on the **Facial Aspect** of a sextant
- Cutting edge C_a is used from disto-facial line angle to midline of the distal surface.
- Cutting edge C_b is used from disto-facial line angle to midline of the mesial surface.

The two cutting edges, C_c and C_d, of working end B are used on the **Lingual Aspect** of a sextant
- Cutting edge C_c is used from disto-lingual line angle to midline of the distal surface.
- Cutting edge C_d is used from disto-lingual line angle to midline of the mesial surface.

STEPS FOR SELECTING THE CORRECT CUTTING EDGE OF A UNIVERSAL CURET IN A POSTERIOR SEXTANT

1. Grasp the instrument in a modified pen grasp and establish a fulcrum.

   Place either working end on a proximal surface apical to the contact area. Establish an appropriate finger rest. Position the handle so it is as parallel as possible to the long axis of the tooth.

   Look closely at the shank nearest the working end. If the lower shank is parallel with the proximal surface, this is the correct cutting edge for this tooth surface.

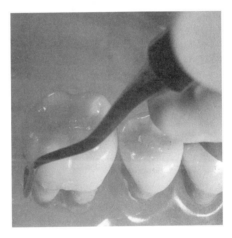

RULE: For posterior teeth, the lower shank should be parallel to the proximal surface.

USE ON POSTERIOR TOOTH SURFACES

Example: Mandibular Right Posteriors, Facial Aspect

1. Select the correct working end of the universal curet.

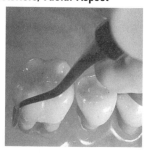

2. The tooth surfaces of the facial aspect should be completed in the order shown in this illustration.

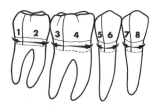

3. Begin with the last molar in the sextant.
   Adapt the leading-third of the cutting edge to the distofacial line angle. The toe of the working end should point toward the back of the mouth because this is the direction in which you are working.

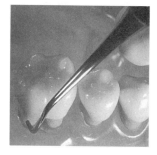

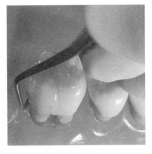

4. Make a series of strokes across the distal surface, ending beneath the contact area.

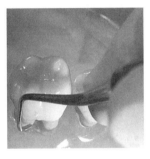

5. While maintaining your fulcrum point, lift the working end away from the tooth and turn the working end so that the toe "points" forward toward the front of the mouth.

    Reposition the cutting edge at the distofacial line angle.

    Activate an oblique working stroke.

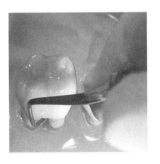

6. If furcation involvement is present, use the leading third of the cutting edge against the mesial surface of the distal root.

7. Continue making a series of oblique strokes across the facial surface.

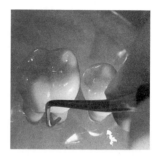

8. Roll the instrument handle slightly to re-adapt the leading third of the cutting edge to the curved root surface.

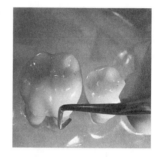

9. At the mesiofacial line angle, roll the handle to readapt the leading third of the cutting edge as you work onto the mesial surface.

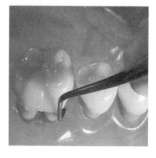

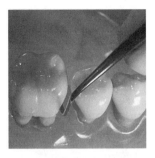

10. Continue making strokes across the mesial surface.

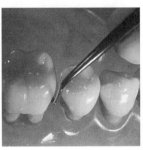

11. Continue strokes until at least 50% of the mesial surface has been instrumented from the facial aspect. The other 50% of the mesial surface will be accessed from the lingual aspect.

MECHANIC'S CHECK

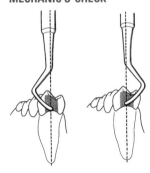

Be sure to extend working strokes past the midline of the proximal surface (i.e., under the contact area) from the facial and lingual aspects.

Section 2:

Use of Area-Specific Curets

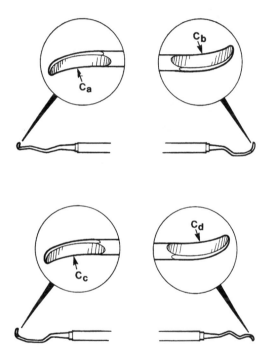

Cutting Edges: Only one cutting edge on each working end of an area-specific curet is used for tooth surface debridement. To complete a posterior sextant, facial and lingual aspects, requires four area-specific curets. For example, Gracey 11, 12, 13, and 14. These curets may be combined on two double-ended instruments.

Facial

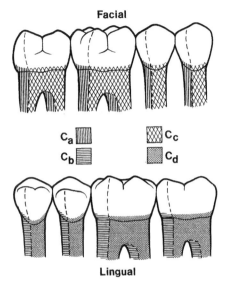

C_a
C_b
C_c
C_d

Lingual

APPLICATION OF AREA-SPECIFIC CURETS TO POSTERIOR TOOTH SURFACES

Cutting edges C_a and C_c are used on the **Facial Aspect** of the sextant:
- Cutting edge C_a is used from disto-facial line angle to midline of the distal surface; then:
- Cutting edge C_c is used from disto-facial line angle to midline of the mesial surface,

Cutting edges C_b and C_d are used on the **Lingual Aspect** of the sextant:
- Cutting edge C_b is used from disto-lingual line angle to midline of the distal surface,
- Cutting edge C_d is used from disto-lingual line angle to midline of the mesial surface.

SELECTING THE CORRECT CUTTING EDGE

STEPS FOR SELECTING THE CORRECT CUTTING EDGE OF A POSTERIOR AREA-SPECIFIC CURET

1. Randomly select one of the posterior area-specific curets for use on the distal surface. For example, use either a Gracey 13 or 14. Grasp the instrument in a modified pen grasp, and establish a fulcrum.

2. Place either working end on a proximal surface.

   Look closely at the shank nearest the working end of the instrument. If the lower shank is parallel to the proximal surface, this is the correct cutting edge for this tooth surface.

RULE: The lower shank should be parallel to the proximal surface.

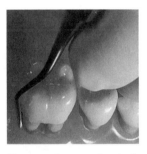

Correct: Lower shank is parallel to the proximal surface—this is the correct cutting edge.

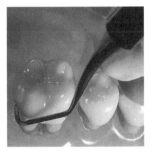

Incorrect: Lower shank is not parallel to the proximal surface—this is the incorrect cutting edge for this tooth surface.

USE ON POSTERIOR TOOTH SURFACES

Example: Mandibular Right Posteriors, Facial Aspect

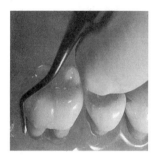

1. Select the correct area-specific curet for use on the distal surface.

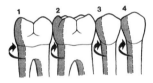

2. The distal surfaces of the facial aspect should be completed in the order shown in this illustration. Remember that different curets will be used on the facial and mesial surfaces.

3. Begin with the last molar in the sextant. Adapt the leading-third of the cutting edge to the distofacial line angle. The toe of the working end should point toward the back of the mouth because this is the direction in which you are working.

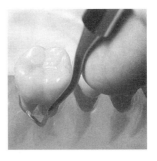

4. Roll the instrument handle to maintain adaptation as you re-position the working end on the distal surface. Make a series of strokes across the distal surface ending beneath the contact area.

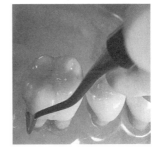

5. Instrument the distal surface of the mesial root with the distal curet.

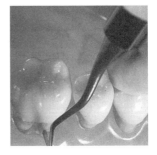

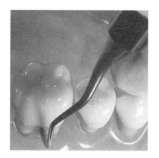

6. Make a series of short vertical strokes along the distal surface of the root.

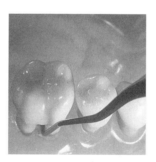

7. Extend the working end as far into the furcation as possible.

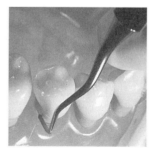

8. Slide your fulcrum point slightly forward in the mouth. Lift the working end away from the tooth, and reposition it on the distal line angle of the next tooth in the sextant. Complete the distal surfaces of each posterior tooth from the facial aspect.

9. Select the correct cu-
    ret for use on the fa-
    cial surfaces. Com-
    plete the facial and
    mesial surfaces in the
    order shown in this
    illustration.

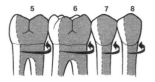

10. Reposition the cut-
    ting edge at the disto-
    facial line angle with
    the toe "pointing"
    forward, toward the
    front of the mouth.
    Activate an oblique
    working stroke.

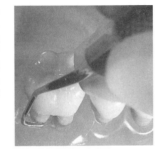

11. If furcation involve-
    ment is present, use
    the curet against the
    mesial surface of the
    distal root.

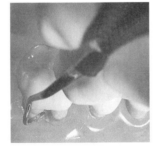

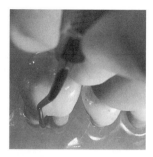

12. Extend the working end as far into the furcation as possible.

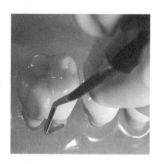

13. Reposition the working end for the facial surface of the mesial root.

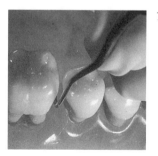

14. At the mesiofacial line angle, roll the handle to readapt the leading-third of the cutting edge as you work onto the mesial surface. Use the mesial curet to instrument the mesial surface of the tooth.

15. Continue strokes until at least 50% of the mesial surface has been instrumented from the facial aspect. The other 50% of the mesial surface will be accessed from the lingual aspect.

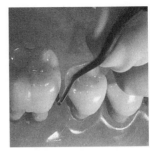

16. Complete the facial and mesial surfaces of the facial aspect for the remaining teeth in the sextant.

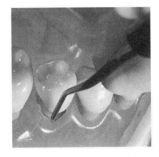

Section 3:

Root Surface Debridement

MECHANIC'S CHECK: INSTRUMENTING MULTI-ROOTED TEETH

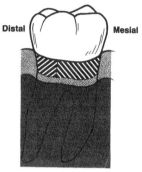

Root trunk:
Cutting edge /// = disto-facial line angle to the distal surface
Cutting edge \\\ = facial and mesial surface of aspect

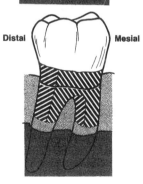

Root Branches: Debride each root as if it was the root of a single-rooted tooth.
Cutting edge /// = distal half of the root
Cutting edge \\\ = mesial half of the root

ROOT MORPHOLOGY REVIEW: POSTERIOR TEETH

Mandibular First Premolar

Mesial surface: depression in cervical area of root; deep linear concavity running length of root

Distal surface: depression in cervical area of root; shallow linear concavity running length of root

Mandibular Second Premolar

Mesial surface of root: shallow depression in cervical area of root; shallow linear concavity sometimes present

Distal surface of root: shallow depression in cervical area of root; usually no linear root concavity

Maxillary First Premolar

Maxillary First Premolar

Mesial surface of root: shallow depression at cervical third; deep linear concavity running from the crown to bifurcation

Furcation: begins in middle- or apical-third of root

Distal surface of root: shallow depression at cervical third; linear concavity running from the cervical line to the bifurcation (less pronounced than concavity on mesial)

Furcation: begins in middle- or apical-third of root

Maxillary Second Premolar

Maxillary Second Premolar

Mesial surface of root: shallow depression at cervical third; shallow linear concavity extending the entire length of the root

Distal surface of root: shallow depression at cervical third; shallow linear concavity extending the entire length of the root

Mandibular First Molar

Mandibular First Molar

Buccal surface of the root trunk: deep depression on root trunk extending from bifurcation to cervical line; depression becomes more shallow toward cervical line

Furcation: 3 mm from cervical line

Lingual surface of the root trunk: deep depression on root trunk extending from bifurcation to cervical line; depression becomes more shallow toward cervical line

Furcation: 3 to 4 mm from cervical line

Mandibular First Molar

Mandibular First Molar

Mesial surface of crown: shallow depression apical to contact area of crown

Mesial surface of root: wide shallow concavity extending the entire length of root

Distal surface of crown: shallow depression apical to contact area of crown

Distal surface of root: wide shallow concavity extending the entire length of root; concavity is less pronounced than the mesial root concavity

Mandibular Second Molar

Root depressions and concavities are similar to those of the mandibular first molar. Furcation is similar to that of the mandibular first molar.

Maxillary First Molar

Buccal surface of root trunk: deep depression extending from bifurcation to cervical line

Furcation: 4 mm from cervical line

Maxillary First Molar

Lingual root: longitudinal groove extending the length of the lingual surface

Furcation: none

Maxillary First Molar

Cervical area of crown: shallow depression on mesial crown surface

Mesial surface of root trunk: deep depression extending from bifurcation to cervical line

Furcation is 4 mm from cervical line; furcation is located closer to the lingual aspect than the facial aspect. Access to furcation is easier from the lingual aspect.

Mesio-buccal root: longitudinal groove on mesial surface

Maxillary First Molar

Cervical area of crown: shallow depression on distal crown surface

Distal surface of root trunk: deep depression extending from bifurcation to cervical line

Furcation is 4 to 5 mm from cervical line.

Disto-buccal root: longitudinal groove on distal surface

MULTIDIRECTIONAL STROKES

Light, multidirectional work strokes are used to remove residual calculus granules and bacterial byproducts from the surface of the cementum. Multidirectional strokes are achieved by employing all three stroke directions, one-by-one in succession.

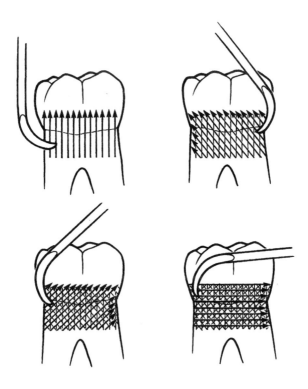

PATTERN OF INSTRUMENTATION STROKES

Most root surface debridement is done beneath the gingival margin. It is important to instrument every millimeter of root surface for de-plaquing, calculus removal, and disruption of endotoxins. Covering every square millimeter of root surface is a challenging task because the clinician usually is working subgingivally and cannot see the tooth surface. In the case of subgingival instrumentation, the clinician must adopt a systematic pattern of instrumentation strokes. A haphazard pattern of strokes will result in sections not being instrumented and unsuccessful treatment of the tooth.

It is helpful to think of the root surface as being divided into a series of long narrow sections or tracts. Each tract is only as wide as the leading-third of the instrument's cutting edge. Begin at the base of the pocket in Tract 1 covering every millimeter from the pocket base to the cementoenamel junction. When Tract 1 is completed, move to Tract 2 and so on.

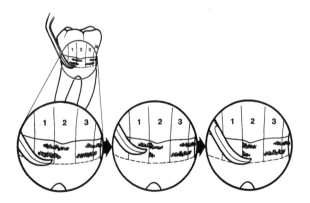

Section 4:

Problem Identification—Difficulties in Instrumentation of Posterior Teeth

Problem	Causes Listed in order from most to least likely cause for each problem
A. Difficulty obtaining vision of posterior teeth	1. Positioning: patient chair is too high in relationship to the seated clinician, causing the clinician to raise shoulders and arms to reach the treatment area. 2. Positioning: patient's head is not in the correct position for the treatment area (i.e., chin up or down, turned toward or away). 3. Positioning: top of patient's head is not even with the top edge of the headrest causing the clinician to stretch (when seated behind patient) in order to reach treatment area. 4. Positioning: clinician is not in the appropriate operator position for surfaces. 5. Mirror is not used, especially for lingual or distal surfaces. 6. Fulcrum: finger rest is too close to the surface being instrumented so the visibility and or activation are restricted. 7. Fulcrum: clinician's hand is blocking the line of vision (could be either mirror hand or instrument hand). 8. Parallelism of lower shank/handle: clinician fails to take the height of contour into consideration when working on cervical-third of crown or on the root; this may result from a lack of skill in using indirect vision.

continued

Problem	Causes Listed in order from most to least likely cause for each problem
B. Difficulty obtaining illumination of a posterior treatment area	1. Positioning: unit light is too near the patient, resulting in excessive shadowing. 2. Positioning: unit light is not directed properly for the arch. 3. Positioning: patient's head is improperly positioned. 4. Mirror: clinician is not using a mirror to reflect light.
C. Difficulty gaining access to a tooth surface with the instrument working end	1. Most likely causes are listed under **Problem A.** 2. Likely causes are listed under **Problem B.** 3. Retraction is inadequate. 4. Grasp: incorrect technique is used with grasp.
D. Incomplete calculus removal	1. Mirror: clinician is not using indirect vision for distal surfaces. 2. Basic concept: clinician is not using any basic skill, such as position, grasp, fulcrum, activation, and adaptation. 3. Design: clinician is not selecting an appropriate instrument for the location or type of calculus. 4. Working end: clinician is not selecting the correct working end and/or cutting edge for surface. 5. Parallelism: lower shank is not parallel to surface being instrumented. 6. Grasp: middle finger is not on the shank, causing the clinician to have limited tactile information. 7. Grasp: clinician is holding the instrument with excessive pressure.

continued

Problem	Causes Listed in order from most to least likely cause for each problem
	8. Adaptation: middle-third of cutting edge is adapted instead of the leading-third of cutting edge. 9. Angulation: clinician has incorrect working angulation. 10. Stroke: clinician is not using light assessment stroke; the clinician's grasp must be relaxed and the stroke must be sweeping to detect irregularities. 11. Visualization: clinician is not establishing a clear mental picture of the location and/or extent of subgingival deposits. 12. Visualization: clinician is trying to actually see subgingival deposits rather than feel them. 13. Stroke: clinician is not applying lateral pressure with index finger or thumb against handle to engage cutting edge against the tooth surface. 14. Stroke: clinician is not overlapping working strokes and working in narrow instrumentation tracts. 15. Detection aid: clinician is not using compressed air or explorer.
E. Calculus deposits missed on proximal surfaces	1. Refer to causes listed under **Problem D.** 2. Adaptation: clinician is not making small continuous adjustments in adaptation while working around the line angle. 3. Adaptation: clinician is not extending the working strokes at least halfway across the proximal surface from the facial and lingual aspects of the tooth.

continued

Problem	Causes Listed in order from most to least likely cause for each problem
	4. Adaptation: clinician is not rolling instrument handle to direct leading-third of cutting edge into root concavities on proximal root surfaces. 5. Stroke: clinician is not applying pressure forward against a distal proximal surface with the cutting edge; clinician is activating stroke in the interproximal space instead of against the tooth. 6. Stroke: clinician is not applying pressure back against a mesial proximal surface with the cutting edge; clinician is activating stroke in the interproximal space instead of against the tooth.
F. Calculus deposits missed at midline region of posterior tooth	1. Refer to causes listed under **Problem D.** 2. Stroke direction: clinician is not using a circumferential (i.e., horizontal) stroke at the midline on facial or lingual aspect of the root surface. 3. Adaptation: clinician is not directing leading-third of cutting edge into root depressions at midline of the facial and lingual aspects of molar teeth or not using horizontal strokes.
G. Calculus deposits missed at line angle region of posterior tooth	1. Refer to causes listed under **Problem D.** 2. Stroke direction: clinician is not using a circumferential (i.e., horizontal) stroke on the line angle region. 3. Adaptation: clinician is not making small continuous adjustments in adaptation while making oblique strokes in the area of the line angle.

continued

Problem	Causes Listed in order from most to least likely cause for each problem
H. Interdental papillae lacerated	1. Handle roll: clinician is not reestablishing adaptation of the leading-third of the cutting edge in the line angle region of the tooth. 2. Adaptation: clinician is attempting to adapt too much of the cutting edge to the tooth in the area of the line angle.
I. Poor tactile discrimination	1. Grasp: clinician's middle finger is not resting lightly on the shank. 2. Grasp: clinician is holding the handle too tightly ("death grip"). 3. Grasp: clinician's index finger and thumb are not opposite each other on the handle. A common problem is holding the index finger on the midsection of handle, whereas the thumb and middle finger are actually being used to hold the instrument. 4. Stroke: clinician does not cover every square millimeter of tooth surface. 5. Strokes: clinician does not extend strokes at least halfway across a proximal surface from the facial and lingual aspects. 6. Strokes: clinician does not begin stroke from the base of pocket.
J. Lack of strength or control with work stroke	1. Grasp: the instrument handle is supported by only the pads of the index finger and thumb in a "pinching" type of grasp. The midsection of the handle does not rest against the side of the index finger or in the "V" of the hand for support.

continued

Problem	Causes Listed in order from most to least likely cause for each problem
	2. Grasp: fingers are spread apart, especially when the fulcrum finger is not in contact with the middle finger, so that the hand is not functioning as a unit. 3. Fulcrum finger: ring finger does not maintain pressure against the rest point on the tooth throughout the stroke; ring finger may actually lift away from its resting point on the tooth; this problem is often seen in combination with point 4 below. 4. Fulcrum finger: ring finger is limp and therefore does not act as the "support beam for the hand" during the stroke. 5. Fulcrum: rest point is too far away or too close to the tooth being instrumented for the size of this clinician's hands and length of fingers. 6. Finger rest: rest is not stable. 7. Advanced fulcruming techniques: clinician attempts using advanced techniques when he or she has not mastered the use of fundamental techniques. 8. Position: clinician has arm pressed against his or her torso so that the arm or wrist motion is restricted. 9. Activation: clinician does not apply lateral pressure to engage cutting edge on tooth with calculus removal stroke. 10. Activation: work strokes are too long or too rapid, causing loss of control.

continued

Problem	Causes Listed in order from most to least likely cause for each problem
	11. Activation: forceful scraping stroke is applied in apical and coronal directions; clinician does not relax strokes when repositioning working end.
K. Inability to obtain adaptation of cutting edge to surface	1. Most common cause is inability to gain access to area—refer to **Problem C.** 2. Inability to obtain vision of the treatment area—refer to **Problem A.** 3. Adaptation: clinician is attempting to adapt too much of the length of the cutting edge to the tooth surface. 4. Instrument design: clinician does not select an appropriate instrument for the task. 5. Also refer to **Problem L** for difficulties in maintaining adaptation.

continued

Problem	Causes Listed in order from most to least likely cause for each problem

L. Difficulties maintaining adaptation	1. Refer to **Problem K** if the problem regards attaining adaptation.
	2. Grasp: imprecise grasp makes it difficult for the clinician to maintain adaptation, especially when:
	  a) the index finger and thumb are not opposite each other on the handle. A common problem is holding the index finger on the midsection of handle so that the thumb and middle finger are actually being used to hold the instrument. This grasp makes it difficult to roll the handle, and it greatly diminishes tactile sensitivity because the middle finger is not on the shank.
	  b) the clinician fails to reposition fingers slightly on handle after rolling it, thus fingers become "tangled up" or "wrapped around each other."
	3. Parallelism in mesial-distal plane: clinician does not keep lower shank parallel to the surface being instrumented.
	4. Parallelism in labial-lingual plane: clinician does not keep lower shank parallel to the surface being instrumented.

Section 5:

References and Suggested Readings

Also refer to References and Suggested Readings for Chapters 3, 4, and 6.

Aoki, A., Ando, Y., Watanabe, H., Ishikawa, I.: In vitro studies on laser scaling of subgingival calculus with an erbium:YAG laser. J Periodontol Dec;65(12):1097-106, 1994.

Ash, M.: Wheeler's dental anatomy, physiology and occlusion. Philadelphia, PA: W.B. Saunders, 1993.

Bower, R.C.: Furcation morphology relative to periodontal treatment. Furcation entrance architecture. J Periodontol Jan;50(1):23-7, 1979.

Bower, R.C.: Furcation morphology relative to periodontal treatment. Furcation root surface anatomy. J Periodontol Jul;50(7):366-74, 1979.

Brand, R., Isselhard, D.: Anatomy of orofacial structures. St. Louis, MO: C.V. Mosby Co., 1990.

Dunlap, R.M., Gher, M.E.: Root surface measurements of the mandibular first molar. J Periodontol Apr;56(4):234-8, 1985.

Gher, M.W. Jr., Dunlap, R.W.: Linear variation of the root surface area of the maxillary first molar. J Periodontol Jan;56(1):39-43, 1985.

Hou, G.L., Tsai, C.C.: Types and dimensions of root trunk correlating with diagnosis of molar furcation involvements. J Clin Periodontol Feb;24(2):129-35, 1997.

Hou, G.L., Chen, S.F., Wu, Y.M., Tsai, C.C.: The topography of the furcation entrance in Chinese molars. Furcation entrance dimensions. J Clin Periodontol Aug;21(7):451-6, 1994.

Hou, G.L., Tsai, C.C.: Relationship between palato-radicular grooves and localized periodontitis. J Clin Periodontol Oct;20(9):678-82, 1993.

Joseph, I., Varma, B.R., Bhat, K.M.: Clinical significance of furcation anatomy of the maxillary first premolar: a biometric study on extracted teeth. J Periodontol Apr;67(4):386-9, 1996.

Marklund, M., Persson, M.: The relationship between mandibular morphology and apical root curvature in man. Arch Oral Biol;33(6):391-4, 1988.

Pecora, J.D., Saquy, P.C., Sousa Neto, M.D., Woelfel, J.B.: Root form and canal anatomy of maxillary first premolars. Braz Dent J;2(2):87-94, 1992.

Sterrett, J.D., Pelletier, H., Russell, C.M.: Tooth thickness at the furcation entrance of lower molars. J Clin Periodontol Jul;23(7):621-7, 1996.

Varrela, J.: Root morphology of mandibular premolars in human 45,X females. Arch Oral Biol;35(2):109-12, 1990.

Walker, RT.: Root form and canal anatomy of mandibular first molars in a southern Chinese population. Endod Dent Traumatol Feb;4(1):19-22, 1988.

Walker, RT.: Root form and canal anatomy of mandibular second molars in a southern Chinese population. J Endod Jul;14(7):325-9, 1988.

6

Mechanized Instruments

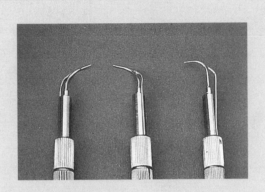

In this chapter

Section 1:

Introduction to Mechanized Instruments

Introduced in the late 1950's, the first mechanized instruments had working ends that were large in size and limited in adaptation. Throughout the 1960's, 70's, and early 80's, ultrasonic and sonic scalers were used primarily for gross calculus removal, followed by hand-activated instruments for definitive instrumentation. In the late 1980's, thin working ends, significantly smaller than the standard Gracey curet, were developed. Modern mechanized instruments are as effective as hand instruments in removing bacterial plaque, plaque retentive supra- and subgingival calculus deposits, and bacterial endotoxins. In addition, these instruments efficiently remove extrinsic stains and orthodontic cement. The 1996 World Workshop in Periodontics review of nonsurgical periodontal instrumentation states that the best instrumentation results are probably achieved by the combined use of mechanized and hand-activated instrumentation.

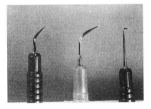

Ultrasonic inserts with large-sized working ends are limited to supragingival use. Shown here are Cavitron ultrasonic inserts (from left to right): Thin Beavertail, 10 Straight, and the 7 Fine-Tipped insert.

Modern ultrasonic inserts with thin working ends provide access to deep periodontal pockets. Shown here are the Cavitron Focused Spray Slimline inserts (from left to right): Slimline (Right), Slimline (Straight), and Slimline (Left).

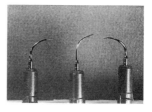

ADVANTAGES

Mechanized instrumentation has several advantages over hand-activated instrumentation. Advantages include: mechanisms of action, design features, and techniques for use.

Mechanisms of Action

While hand instruments mechanically clean the tooth surface, mechanized instruments combine three mechanisms: (1) mechanical, (2) fluid lavage, and (3) acoustic turbulence.

Mechanical action: mechanized instruments use an instrument tip, vibrating at a high-frequency, to remove bacterial plaque, plaque retentive calculus deposits, and endotoxins from the tooth surface.

Fluid lavage: a constant stream of fluid runs through the handpiece of a mechanized instrument and exits near the instrument tip. This stream of fluid produces a **flushing action** that washes calculus debris, bacteria, and unattached plaque from the treatment site. The flushing action removes blood and debris from the site, which allows better vision during instrumentation.

Acoustic turbulence: the pressure produced by the continuous stream of fluid flowing into the confined space of the periodontal pocket is known as "acoustic turbulence." Bacteria and gram-negative motile rods, in particular, are sensitive to acoustic energy. Acoustic turbulence has an **antimicrobial effect** within the environment of the pocket. Sites debrided with mechanized instruments have lower levels of bacteria than sites instrumented by hand.

Design Features

Size of the Instrument Working End: The working end of a thin mechanized instrument tip is significantly smaller in size than the working end of a hand-activated curet. Standard Gracey curets are too wide to enter the furcation area of more than 50% of all maxillary and mandibular molars. The curet cutting-edge must be adapted at a 70° to 80° angle to the tooth surface; placement of the instrument can result in significant tissue displacement. The thin mechanized instrument tip is positioned in much the same manner as a periodontal probe, causing little tissue displacement.

Active Portion of the Working End: The last 2 to 4 millimeters of a mechanized instrument tip are active; both sides, and in some cases, the back and face of the working end can be used for debridement. With a hand-activated instrument, only the cutting edge is capable of doing work.

Handpiece Design: One of the most stressful elements of instrumentation is the pinch pressure used to grasp the instrument handle. Mechanized instruments have large diameter handpieces that require less pinch pressure to hold.

Thin ultrasonic tips are similar in size to calibrated periodontal probes. Thin tips with an extended shank design provide excellent accessibility for debridement of periodontal pockets.

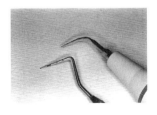

Techniques for Use

Grasp and Stroke Pressure: Mechanized instruments use high-frequency vibrations rather than the clinician's muscle power for debridement. These instruments can be used with a light, relaxed grasp and light stroke pressure.

Shorter Instrumentation Time: Significantly less time is needed to accomplish debridement with mechanical instruments. The ergonomic advantages of less pinch pressure, a relaxed grasp, and light stroke pressure combined with shorter instrumentation time are important advantages of mechanical debridement.

Less Iatrogenic Damage to Periodontium:

Tissue Healing. Mechanized instruments have no cutting edges to cut or tear the tissue; this is especially helpful when working in deep, confined pocket areas. Less tissue trauma results in faster healing rates for sites treated with mechanized instruments.

Minimal Cementum Removal. A thin mechanized instrument tip will remove less cementum and, therefore, provides the most conservative approach to subgingival debridement. Conservation of cementum is advantageous to periodontal health. Research studies indicate that thin-sized mechanized tips remove the least amount of cementum, hand-activated curets remove a moderate amount of cementum, and large-sized mechanized tips remove the most cementum.

Glossary of Terms

MECHANIZED INSTRUMENTS

Ultrasonics are devices operating at frequencies above the audible range. In dentistry, this includes systems in the 18,000 to 50,000 cycles per second (cps) (18 to 50 kilohertz [kHz]) range.

Sonics are devices operating in the audible range. Current sonic units operate at 3,000 to 8,000 cps (3 to 8 kHz).

FREQUENCY

Frequency is the number of times per second the instrument tip moves back and forth during one cycle (excursion).

Cycle is one complete linear or elliptical stroke path of tip.

Kilohertz (kHz) is equal to 1000 hertz, or 1000 cps.

Active Tip Area is the portion of the instrument tip that is capable of doing work. Active tip area is affected by frequency. In the 25,000 to 30,000 cps, the active tip area is approximately 4.3 mm. In the 40,000 to 50,000 cps, the active tip area is less than 2.4 mm.

TUNING

Auto tuning: The tip frequency is controlled automatically by the system.

Manual Tuning: On ultrasonic units, the tip frequency is adjusted by the clinician using the tuning knob.

POWER

Power is the energy in the handpiece used to generate the movement of the insert. Increasing the power increases the distance the instrument tip moves (i.e., length of the work stroke).

Stroke is the maximum distance the instrument tip moves during one cycle. On ultrasonic units, the stroke is adjusted by the power knob.

Load is the resistance on an instrument tip when placed against the calculus deposit on the tooth surface.

Clinical Power is the ability to remove calculus deposits under load. The stroke, frequency, type of tip motion, and angulation of the motion against the tooth surface are factors that determine clinical power.

Glossary of Terms is courtesy of DENTSPLY Preventive Care Division.

TYPES

The three types of mechanized instruments are magneto (i.e., magnetostrictive) ultrasonic, piezo (i.e., piezoelectric) ultrasonic, and sonic.

Ultrasonic Mechanized Instruments

Ultrasonic mechanized units use an electric current to convert electric signals to mechanical energy in the form of high-frequency vibrations on the instrument tip. There are two types of ultrasonic instruments: magneto and piezo.

The Magneto Ultrasonic Unit (pronounced *mag'-net-oh*)

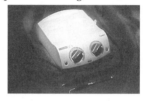

Magneto Ultrasonic Unit. The magneto ultrasonic unit consists of an electric generator housed in a portable cabinet, a handpiece, and interchangeable insert tips. A foot pedal activates power and water for the instrument. (Photograph courtesy of DENTSPLY Preventive Care.)

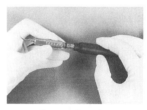

A magneto insert tip. The handpiece of a magneto ultrasonic unit holds interchangeable insert tips.

The Piezo Ultrasonic Unit (pronounced *pee-ay'-zoe*)

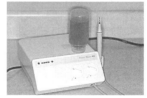

Piezo Ultrasonic Unit. The pictured piezo ultrasonic generator has a self-contained irrigation bottle and pump making it a truly portable system. (Photograph courtesy of Electro Medical Systems.)

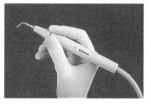

A piezo handpiece with instrument tip.
Instrument tips screw onto the handpiece. A special wrench is used to attach and remove the tips from the handpiece. A foot pedal activates power and water for the instrument. (Photograph courtesy of Electro Medical Systems.)

Sonic Mechanized Instruments

Sonic mechanized instruments use compressed air to power a turbine at high rotational speeds, resulting in low-frequency vibrations of the instrument tip.

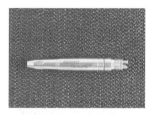

The sonic handpiece.
The sonic handpiece connects directly to the compressed-air line of the dental unit.

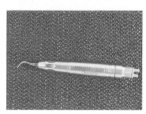

A sonic handpiece and instrument tip.
The instrument tips screw onto the handpiece. A special wrench is used to attach and remove the tips from the handpiece. The dental unit rheostat activates the instrument.

CONTRAINDICATIONS FOR USE

With all of the benefits of mechanized instruments, it is important to remember that these instruments are not recommended for use with all patients. Mechanized instrumentation is not recommended for patients with communicable diseases, patients with an increased susceptibility to infection, pediatric patients, and patients with certain dental conditions.

The use of ultrasonic or sonic instruments is contraindicated for patients with

1. Communicable diseases that can be disseminated by aerosols (e.g., hepatitis, tuberculosis, Strep throat, flu, and respiratory infections).
2. High susceptibility to opportunistic infections that can be transmitted by contaminated dental-unit water or aerosols (e.g., patients with uncontrolled diabetes, debilitated patients with chronic medical conditions, or immuno-suppressed patients [i.e., organ-transplant recipients; patients with cancer, systemic lupus erythematosus, or Crohn's disease; and patients who are HIV-positive or who meet the "Rule of Twos" for cortico-steroid use]).
3. Respiratory or pulmonary disease or who experience difficulty breathing. These patients would be at high risk for infection if they were to aspirate microorganisms from plaque into the lungs.
4. Certain styles of cardiac pacemaker because they may be effected by magneto instruments; newer pacemakers have built in shields that make ultrasonic instrumentation safe. Check with a cardiologist.
5. Compromised or lessened gag reflex or difficulties in swallowing.
6. Certain dental conditions (i.e., porcelain crowns, composite resin restoration, demineralized enamel surfaces, and dentinal sensitivity). Porcelain and composite resin restorations can be damaged by mechanized instruments; avoid contact of working end with these restorations. Not for use with titanium implants, unless the ultrasonic instrument is covered with a specially designed plastic sleeve.
7. Young, growing tissue. Vibrations may damage growing tissues in children.
8. Primary and newly erupted teeth because these teeth have large pulp chambers that are more susceptible to heat generated by instruments.

PREVENTION OF BIOFILM CONTAMINATION IN DENTAL UNIT WATERLINES

Scientific studies have shown that dental unit waterlines may become significantly contaminated with microorganisms including Staphylococcus, Legionella, Pseudomonas, and Moraxella. This microbial contaminated water is delivered to ultrasonic/sonic mechanized instruments, dental handpieces, and air/water syringes. Although water from a municipal water source is safe for drinking, the presence of even small numbers of organisms can present problems for dental unit water quality. Potable drinking water is defined as less than 500 bacterial colony–forming units per milliliter (CFU/ml). Water recovered from dental units connected to municipal water supplies may contain millions of bacterial CFU/ml.

Patients at Risk

Patients at risk of iatrogenic infection linked to dental treatment include: the elderly; patients with chronic medical conditions or diabetes; patients who smoke or suffer from alcoholism or are immuno-suppressed (i.e., organ-transplant recipients or patients with cancer) or HIV-positive. Patients and clinicians temporarily compromised by infections and stress also may be at risk of infection.

Biofilms are microbial accumulations that adhere to the interior surfaces of waterline tubing. These biofilms have been shown to be the primary source of contaminated water delivered by dental units. Stagnant water at room temperature is an ideal culture medium for many microorganisms. Dental tubing presents a favorable environment for bacterial colonization because fluid flow is practically stagnant near the tubing walls. Stagnant fluid flow allows floating bacteria to form organized, intricate colonies on the tubing walls. These bacterial colonies are embedded in a polysaccharide slime layer that protects the bacteria from physical or chemical destruction. Parts of the biofilm frequently disengage from the tubing walls and can be carried into the patient's mouth.

Organisms in the structure of a biofilm are highly resistant to chemical germicides and, therefore, act as a source for the continuous recontamination of dental unit water. Improving the quality of dental water is a growing concern for dental healthcare providers striving to maintain high quality patient care. The medical risk from the microbial contamination of dental water is most significant to immune-deficient patients.

Current designs of dental unit waterlines are incapable of delivering water of an optimal microbiologic quality. In a statement on dental unit waterlines on December 13, 1995, the ADA Council on Scientific Affairs encouraged the industry and research community to improve the design of dental equipment by the year 2000. The Council's goal is that water delivered to patients during nonsurgical dental procedures will contain no more than 200 CFU/ml of aerobic mesophilic heterotrophic bacteria in the unfiltered output of the dental unit. This level of bacterial CFU is equivalent to the quality assurance standard for fluid delivery systems in hemodialysis units.

At the present time, the ADA recommends that dental offices employ a combination of strategies for improving dental unit water quality. Commercially available options to control microbial contamination of dental water include:

1. Self-contained water reservoir systems—some reservoir systems allow heat sterilization of all the system's components, including, water bottles, tubing, and control box. Sterilization for 60 minutes at 125° and 20 psi, or 10 minutes at 134° and 30 psi, is recommended.
2. Point-of-use filters for installation in dental unit waterlines may physically reduce the numbers of microorganisms that progress into the output water for handpieces and mechanized instruments. The microfiltration cartridges snap into the waterline and are changed daily to ensure efficacy.
3. Chemical disinfection protocols, daily draining, and air purging regimens

Point-of-use filters are installed in dental unit waterlines to minimize the delivery of contaminated water to the patient's mouth by the mechanized instruments, dental handpieces, and air/water syringes.

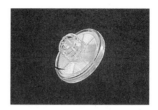

These filters are easily installed in existing dental unit waterlines. Pictured here is the 0.2 micron CLEARLINE filter from Sultan Chemists, Inc.

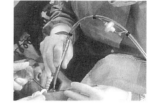

Section 2:

Techniques for Use

Equipment Selection and Infection Control

Equipment Selection	When purchasing equipment, look for a selection of varied instrument tip designs, including thin and furcation tips.
Instrument Selection	Just as with hand-activated instruments, select the appropriate tip for the task at hand. Larger, stronger tips should be used for heavy calculus removal; thin tips should be used for light deposits, de-plaquing, and removal of endotoxins from the surface of the cementum.
Condition of Equipment	Monitor the condition of the equipment. Replace a tip as soon as it shows signs of wear or damage; use manufacturer wear indicators to monitor wear. Thin tips need to be replaced more frequently than larger tips. Use of worn tips can result in damage to the tooth surface. Check the metal stacks on the magneto insert tip; if the magneto insert tip does not slide freely into the handpiece, the tip will not function effectively.
Water Control	Use a disposable high-volume evacuation tip for suction. Water control reduces aerosol production, improves visibility of the treatment area, and increases patient comfort.

continued

Infection Control	Aerosols produced may be contaminated with pathogens. Ultrasonic and sonic instruments produce a high level of aerosol contamination in the dental operatory. Use of barriers, surface disinfection, protective clothing, and laminar airflow systems are recommended. Independent water reservoirs or point-of-use filters are recommended to reduce the number of microorganisms in the water. Patients should rinse with an antimicrobial solution before starting an ultrasonic or sonic procedure. Pretreatment with an antimicrobial rinse reduces the number of airborne microorganisms in aerosols created by water spray. Pre-procedural subgingival irrigation and rinsing can significantly reduce the level of bacteremia associated with ultrasonic scaling.
Personal Protection	Clinicians should use recommended personal protection gear: gown with high neck and long sleeves, hair covering, a high bacterial filtration efficiency (HBFE) face mask, protective eyewear, face shield, and gloves. The face mask should be changed every 20 minutes because a damp mask does not provide adequate protection.
Patient Protection	Personal protection gear for the patient includes: a plastic drape, towel or bib, and protective eyewear. The patient may prefer to cover the nose with a flat-style face mask to limit inhalation of aerosols.

FLUID LAVAGE

Water Flow to the Working End

This mechanized instrument tip has an external water flow tube to carry water to the instrument tip. The water breaks into a fine mist near the end of the external flow tube and at high power settings at the end of the tip.

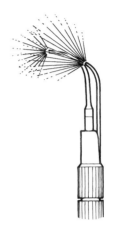

This mechanized instrument tip has an internal water flow system. The water flows directly through the instrument tip, and at high power settings, breaks into a fine mist at the end of the tip.

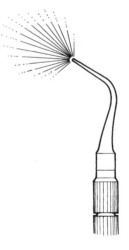

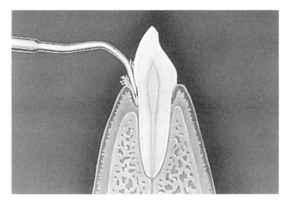

Thin ultrasonic instrument tips are able to carry water (or fluid solutions) to the base of a periodontal pocket. (Illustration courtesy of DENTSPLY Preventive Care.)

Delivery of Solution from an Independent Fluid Reservoir

The fluid irrigant solution used most often with mechanical instruments is tap water. Some ultrasonic units have independent reservoirs that can be used to deliver other fluid solutions to the mechanized instrument tip. Solutions commonly used for irrigation include distilled water, sterile saline, stannous fluoride, and antimicrobial solutions, such as chlorhexidine. The independent fluid reservoir allows the clinician to select the fluid solution appropriate for the patient's periodontal health status and the fluid temperature that is most comfortable for the patient.

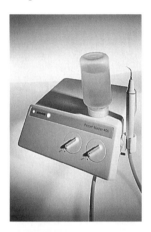

The EMS Piezon Master 400 is an example of a piezo ultrasonic unit with an independent reservoir.

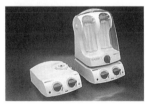

The DENTSPLY SPS Dual Select is an independent reservoir system that can be attached to all Cavitron units.

INSTRUMENTATION TECHNIQUES WITH MECHANIZED INSTRUMENTS

Grasp	Clinician should have a relaxed, light instrument grasp.
Finger Rest	Clinician may use intra- or extra-oral rest. An intraoral fulcrum is not needed to concentrate the force of the stroke because the instrument does the work of mechanical calculus removal. In many cases, an advanced fulcruming technique is advantageous in obtaining access to deep periodontal pockets.
Activation	Digital (i.e., finger) activation is recommended because the instrument is doing the work of calculus removal. Digital activation is excellent for applying the light stroke pressure needed for mechanized instrumentation.
Adaptation of Working End	Position the working end in a manner similar to that of a calibrated periodontal probe, with the point aiming toward the base of the pocket and the length of the working end parallel to the root surface. Adapt the last several millimeters of the side of the working end to the tooth surface. For magneto ultrasonic and sonic instruments, the sides and back of the working end can be used for instrumentation. Instrumentation with the sides of the working end is recommended when using piezo ultrasonic instruments. AVOID direct adaptation of the ''point'' of the working end to the tooth surface.

continued

Power Settings	Use the lowest power setting possible. AVOID high power settings.
Sequence for Calculus Removal	Work in a coronal-to-apical sequence when removing calculus deposits, removing the coronal-most deposits first. This differs from instrumentation with hand instruments where calculus deposits are removed in an apical-coronal sequence.
Stroke Pressure	Use light stroke pressure. It is necessary only to touch the working end to the deposit and allow the mechanized instrument to do all the work. Moderate or heavy stroke pressure actually diminishes the effectiveness of the stroke in some systems.
Stoke Technique	Cover every millimeter of the root surface with overlapping, brushlike strokes.

Instrument Stroke Pattern

Multidirectional, overlapping strokes are used to cover every square millimeter of the root surface. Stroke pressure should be light; the stroke pattern should be long and flowing. The strokes are made in a continuous brushlike manner over the tooth surface. The overlapping strokes should cover every square millimeter of the root surface.

Circumferential Strokes

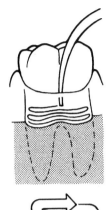

Circumferential stroke on facial or lingual aspect; tip parallel to long axis of tooth.

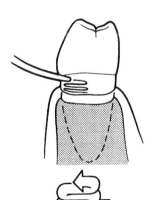

Circumferential stroke on proximal surface with tissue recession present. Tip perpendicular to long axis of tooth.

Vertical Strokes

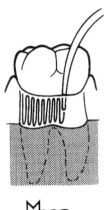

Vertical stroke on facial or lingual aspect; tip parallel to long axis of tooth.

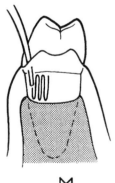

Vertical stroke on proximal aspect; tip parallel to long axis of tooth.

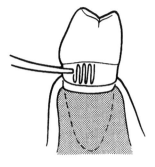

Vertical stroke on proximal surface with tissue recession present. Tip perpendicular to long axis of tooth.

Oblique Strokes

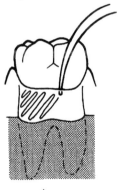

Oblique stroke on facial or lingual aspect; tip angled slightly toward front of mouth.

Oblique stroke on proximal aspect; tip slanted slightly toward facial aspect.

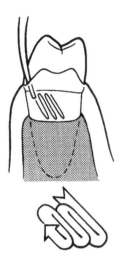

Oblique stroke on proximal surface with tissue recession present; tip slanted slightly toward facial aspect.

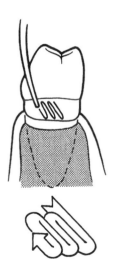

REDUCING AEROSOL PRODUCTION AND BACTEREMIAS

Pre-Procedural Rinsing and Irrigation

In addition to prophylactic antibiotic regimens for patients who are at risk of developing bacterial endocarditis, the American Heart Association now recommends the use of pre-procedural rinsing and subgingival irrigation with an antimicrobial solution. Pre-procedural rinsing and subgingival irrigation with an antimicrobial solution has been shown to significantly reduce the level of blood-borne microorganisms resulting from nonsurgical dental procedures, including instrumentation with mechanized instruments.

Pre-procedural rinsing with either chlorhexidine or an antiseptic mouthrinse, such as Listerine Antiseptic, for 20 to 30 seconds before treatment is recommended for all patients. This procedure is recommended to reduce the number of bacteria introduced into the patient's blood stream and for control of aerosols into the surrounding environment.

Pre-procedural subgingival irrigation of the treatment area with either chlorhexidine or an antiseptic mouthrinse, such as Listerine Antiseptic, is recommended for patients with gingivitis or periodontitis. The antimicrobial solution may be delivered with an irrigating syringe, a subgingival irrigation delivery device (such as a Teledyne Perio Pik), or an ultrasonic unit with a fluid reservoir.

Control of Aerosol Production

Dental procedures disperse airborne particles, called "aerosols," into the surrounding environment. Particles found in dental aerosols include oral microorganisms, blood, saliva, and oral debris. Microorganisms in the dental aerosols have been shown to survive for up to 24 hours.

Ultrasonic and sonic instrumentation have been shown to generate high levels of aerosols. The use of barriers, surface disinfection, and protective attire for the patient and clinician are particularly important when using a mechanized instrument. Laminar airflow systems, which filter microorganisms from the air, are recommended for dental offices.

Control of Water Spray

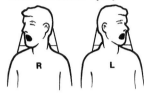

Patient head position. The patient's head should be turned to the right for treatment areas on the right side of the mouth and turned to the left for treatment areas on the left side of the mouth.

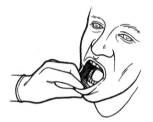

Water control in anterior sextants. Lower and upper lips can be cupped to contain the water spray.

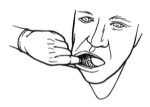

Water control in posterior treatment areas. Hold the cheek between the index finger and thumb, and pull out and up or down to form a cup.

Section 3:

Ultrasonic Instruments

MAGNETO ULTRASONIC INSTRUMENTS		

Examples	Adec (Cavitron)
	Bobcat
	Cavitron SPS, Cavitron
	   Model 3000
	Engler Ultrason 990
	Le Clean Machine
	Maliga Microson 102
		Parkell Turbo 25/30
		Periogiene Odontoson
		Sonatron
		Sonus V
		Southeast Instruments
		   Autoscaler
		USI ultrasonic units

Device	Electronic generator and water control are housed in a portable enclosure. All units permit adjustment of power (stroke) and water. Some units have feedback coils in the handpiece that sense tip motion. The foot control activates power and water flow in all units except the Odontoson, which has a finger-switch activation. Some models have detachable handpieces that are capable of being sterilized, others have only removable sheaths or must be wipe disinfected. All units except Engler 990 and Sonus V accept removable interchangeable ultrasonic inserts. These systems have handpiece-mounted stacks and use screw-on tips. The Odontoson unit accepts only Odontoson ferrite stack inserts.	
Principle	The instrument is comprised of an electronic generator, a handpiece assembly containing a coil to energize the insert, and a variety of interchangeable inserts. The generator produces an alternating low voltage electric current in the handpiece. This current produces a magnetic field in the handpiece that causes the insert to expand and contract along its length and, in turn, causes the insert tip to vibrate.	

continued

Water	Water, or another fluid, such as an antimicrobial solution, is directed onto the tip through a metal flow tube or internal channel through the working end. The primary purposes of water in the magneto systems are to cool the tip-tooth interface and flush the sulcus. The water flow required to cool the magneto handpiece is heated to provide a comfortable lavage temperature. Certain magneto systems, such as Cavitron units, allow antimicrobial solutions to be used instead of water in the coolant system for enhanced elimination of bacteria.
Vibration	Magneto Vibration Frequency: Tip vibration is in the range of 18,000 to 42,000 cps (18–42 kHz).
Tip Motion	Insert tips typically move in a controlled elliptical pattern. All surfaces of the insert tip are active; this means the face, back, and both sides of the working end can be used for instrumentation. The active tip area is approximately 4.2 mm for the 25 and 30 kHz units.

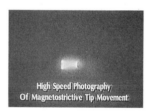

High magnification photography of the elliptical tip movement of a Cavitron magneto mechanized tip.

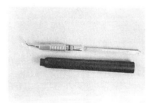

A Cavitron insert tip (top). A wide variety of insert tips are available for Cavitron ultrasonic scalers. The interchangeable inserts are held in a handpiece (bottom).

OPERATION OF MAGNETO ULTRASONIC INSTRUMENTS
Example: DENTSPLY/Cavitron Ultrasonic Scaler

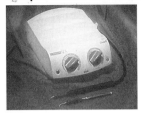

1. Place the ultrasonic power unit on an operatory counter or cart so that you have easy access to the unit and dental chair. (Photographs of operation of Cavitron Ultrasonic Scaler courtesy of DENTSPLY Preventive Care.)

2. Plug the power unit into the electric and water sources. Or if using an independent water reservoir, plug the ultrasonic unit into the electrical outlet, and attach the reservoir bottle. Turn on the dental unit and open water control knob. Flush the dental unit evacuation system with water or cleaning solution for 5 to 10 minutes before the first patient of the day and for 3 to 5 minutes between patients.

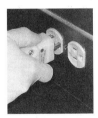 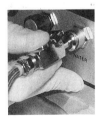

3. Connect a sterilized Steri-Mate handpiece to the handpiece hose. Cover the power unit, and wrap the tubing with a barrier.

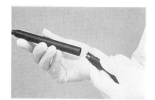

4. Hold the ultrasonic handpiece over a sink. Step on the foot pedal to activate a steady stream of water from the handpiece. Running the water in this manner flushes stagnant water and air from the unit waterlines. At the start of each day, run the water in this manner for 2 minutes. Between patients, run water for 30 seconds.

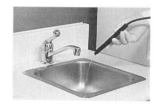

5. Hold handpiece upright, step on foot control, and fill the handpiece completely with water. Keeping the handpiece in an upright position, release foot pedal.

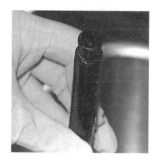

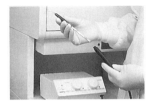

6. Insert a sterilized insert tip into the handpiece, pushing until the insert snaps into place.

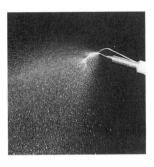

7. Adjust power and water controls while holding the handpiece over the operatory sink. At higher power settings, the water spray should create a light mist or "halo" effect at the working end.

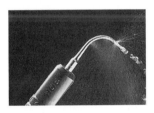

Adjust water control for lower power settings; the water flow should be changed to produce a rapid drip at the working end.

8. Preprocedural rinsing and irrigation. Ask the patient to rinse with an antimicrobial solution for 30 seconds. If appropriate, complete a preprocedural subgingival irrigation of the treatment area before instrumentation.

9. Establish an intra- or extraoral finger rest. Hold the insert tip off of the tooth surface as you step on the control pedal to activate the unit.

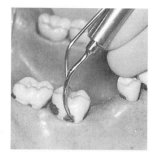

10. Adapt the instrument tip to the tooth surface. Position the tip so the length of the tip is adapted to the tooth surface in a manner similar to that of a calibrated periodontal probe.

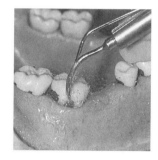

11. Have an assistant use a high-volume suction tip, or, if working alone, ask the patient to hold a saliva ejector. Use light stroke pressure in a sweeping brushlike motion. Use an overlapping multidirectional stroke pattern on each tooth.

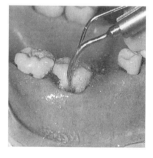

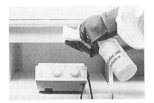

12. **After completion of appointment,** don utility gloves. Remove barriers from equipment, and clean and disinfect equipment.

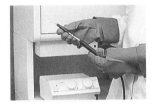

13. Remove the insert tip, and put it aside for processing.

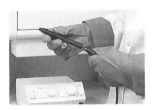

14. Remove the handpiece from the cable, and put it aside for processing.

15. Disinfect the hand-piece connector and tubing using standard infection control procedures.

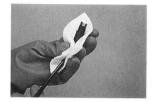

16. Rinse handpiece, and insert tips under running water. Dry thoroughly, and seal in autoclave pouches. Separate pouches should be used for the handpiece and inserts.

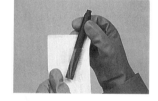

17. Sterilize handpiece and inserts in an autoclave or chemiclave.

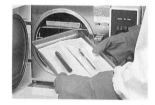

Insert Tip Selection for Magneto Ultrasonic Instruments
Example: DENTSPLY/Cavitron Ultrasonic Scalers

Cavitron Insert Series	Design Characteristics
Classic P	• Standard-sized tips with external water tubes • Designed to operate with vibrations of up to 25 kHZ (cps) • Original insert series first introduced in 1957
Thru Flow (TFI)	• Standard-sized tips with internal water flow (no external water tubes) • Available in 25 kHZ and 30 kHZ designs • First introduced in 1974

continued

Design Characteristics	Cavitron Insert Series
• Thin-sized, probelike tips with external water tubes • Available in 25 kHZ and 30 kHZ designs	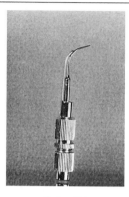 Slimline (SLI)
• Standard-sized tips with an internal water delivery system that delivers water directly to the insert tip • Available in 25 kHZ and 30 kHZ designs	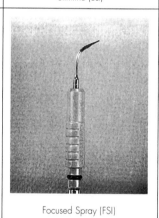 Focused Spray (FSI)

continued

Cavitron Insert Series	Design Characteristics
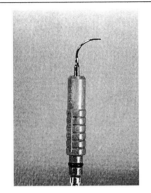 Focused Spray Slimline	• Thin-sized, probelike tips with an internal water delivery system that delivers water directly to the insert tip • Available in 25 kHZ and 30 kHZ designs

Insert Tip Designs

Recommended Use	Cavitron Tip Designs
• Anterior sextants, lingual aspect • Heavy calculus deposits • Supragingival use • Use end of tip; avoid using sides or face of tip.	 3 Thin Beavertail
• Universal use; provides improved access to line angles and interproximal surfaces • Heavy calculus deposits • Supragingival use	 1000 Straight Triple-Bend

continued

Cavitron Tip Designs	Recommended Use
 1 Chisel	• Anterior teeth and premolars • Heavy calculus removal; correcting overhanging margins • Supragingival use
 10 Straight	• Universal use • Moderate calculus deposits • Supragingival or subgingival use where distended tissue allows easy insertion

continued

Recommended Use	Cavitron Tip Designs
• Anterior sextants • Moderate calculus deposits • Supragingival use	 7 Fine-Tipped
• Universal use • Moderate to light calculus deposits • Supragingival use	 Focused Spray 10

Cavitron Tip Designs	Recommended Use
\n\nEWPP Perio-Probe	• Universal use\n• Light calculus deposits and deplaquing\n• Supragingival and subgingival use\n• Use overlapping horizontal and vertical strokes
\n\nSlimline (Straight)	• Set comprised of straight, right, and left insert tips\n• Light calculus removal and deplaquing in shallow pockets\n• Supragingival and subgingival use in shallow pockets\n• Slimline tips come in straight and mirror-image; right/left designs

continued

Recommended Use	Cavitron Tip Designs
<ul><li>Universal use on root surfaces</li><li>Light calculus removal and de-plaquing</li><li>Subgingival use in shallow and deep periodontal pockets</li><li>FSI Slimline tips come in straight and mirror-image; right/left designs</li></ul>	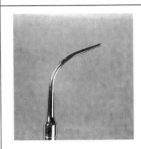 FSI Slimline (Straight)
<ul><li>Root surface concavities and furcation areas</li><li>Light calculus removal and de-plaquing</li><li>Subgingival use in shallow and deep periodontal pockets</li><li>FSI Slimline tips come in straight and mirror-image; right/left designs</li></ul>	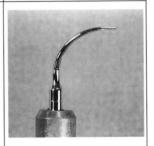 FSI Slimline (Right)

Piezo Ultrasonic Instruments

PIEZO ULTRASONIC INSTRUMENTS		
Examples	Amadent Neosonic-s, Amdent 830 EMS miniPiezon EMS Piezon Master PDT Sensor Sc/RP	Spartan Piezoelectric Ultra Scaler Young PS
Device	Electronic generator and water control are housed in a portable enclosure. All units permit adjustment of power (stroke) and water. The foot control activates power and water flow in all units. Instrument tips screw directly onto the handpiece with the use of a special tool. Tips are not interchangeable from manufacturer to manufacturer. Some models have detachable (autoclavable only) handpieces that are capable of being sterilized, others have only removable sheaths or must be wipe disinfected. Some units have an electronic sensor in the handpiece that can override front panel power settings to lower or boost power.	
Principle	This system is comprised of an electronic generator, a handpiece assembly containing piezo (ceramic) crystals to energize a scaling tip, and a variety of interchangeable screw-on tips. The generator produces an alternating, high voltage in the handpiece. This voltage produces an electric field in the handpiece that causes the piezo crystals to expand and contract along their diameter and, in turn, causes the scaling tip to vibrate.	

continued

Water	The primary purposes of water in the piezo system are to cool the tip-tooth interface and flush the sulcus. Some preheating of the water may be necessary to provide a comfortable lavage temperature. Some systems, such as the EMS Piezon Master, can be used with antimicrobial solutions instead of water for enhanced elimination of bacteria.
Vibrations	Piezo Vibration Frequency: Tip vibration is in the range of 24,000 to 45,000 cps (24–45 kHz).
Tip	Insert tips typically move in a controlled linear pattern. The sides of the working end are recommended for instrumentation. The active tip area varies from approximately 2.2 to 3.5 mm for the 25 and 30 kHz units, depending on tip design.

High magnification photography of the linear tip movement of a piezo-mechanized instrument. (Photograph courtesy of EMS Electro Medical Systems.)

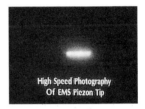

OPERATION OF PIEZO ULTRASONIC INSTRUMENTS

Example: EMS Piezo-Ceramic Ultrasonic Scaler

1. Place the ultrasonic power unit on an operatory counter or cart so that you have easy access to the unit and the dental chair.

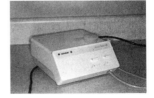

2. Plug the power cord into the back of the ultrasonic unit. Flush the dental unit evacuation system with water or cleaning solution for 5 to 10 minutes before the first patient of the day and for 3 to 5 minutes between patients.

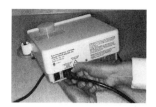

3. If using a unit with a water reservoir, attach the bottle by inserting the sealing disk into the unit and turning it in a clockwise direction for 1/4 turn until the reservoir drops into place. If the reservoir leaks, the red gasket is probably wrinkled; remove the reservoir bottle and straighten the red gasket. If your unit does not have a reservoir, plug the unit water line connection into the water outlet on the dental unit.

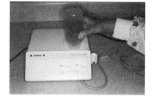

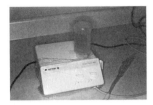

4. Cover the power unit and handpiece hose with barriers. Turn the power unit ON with the switch located on the back of the ultrasonic unit.

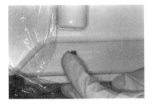

5. Set the power switch on the side of the ultrasonic unit to the SCALING position (rather than the END-ODONTIC position). Hold the handpiece hose over a sink. Step on the foot pedal to activate a steady stream of water from the hose. At the start of the day, run the water in this manner for 2 minutes. Between patients, run the water for 30 seconds.

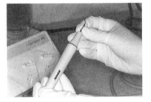

6. Attach handpiece to the handpiece hose. Attach the instrument tip, hand tightening the tip in a clockwise motion.

7. Next, tighten the instrument tip with the autoclutch wrench in a clockwise direction, until you hear a click. When a click is heard, the tip is attached at the proper tightness. The autoclutch wrench protects your fingers when attaching and removing the instrument tips.

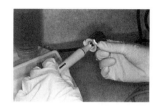

8. Adjust the power setting. For standard calculus removal, begin with the medium power setting (i.e., 10 o'clock on dial) and adjust the setting according to patient sensitivity and the tenacity of the calculus deposits. For subgingival debridement, begin with power and irrigant settings at the 9 o'clock position. When using the thin perio tips, begin with the power setting at 9 o'clock and increase the irrigant setting to at least 11 o'clock.

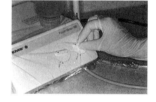

9. Use the water control knob to adjust the irrigant flow to a fine spray. Increase the irrigant flow if heavy calculus deposits require extended treatment in one area.

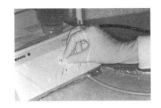

10. Pre-procedural rinsing and irrigation. Ask the patient to rinse with an antimicrobial solution for 30 seconds. If appropriate, complete a pre-procedural subgingival irrigation of the treatment area before instrumentation. Position the patient in a supine position; provide the patient with tissues.

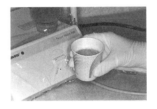

11. Establish an extra- or intraoral finger rest. Hold the instrument tip off of the tooth surface as you step on the foot pedal to activate the instrument.

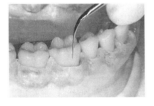

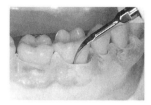

12. The side of the instrument tip is used for instrumentation. Position the tip in a similar manner to a calibrated periodontal probe, with the length of the tip parallel to the long axis of the tooth.

13. Have an assistant use a high-volume suction tip, or, if working alone, ask the patient to hold a saliva ejector. Use light stroke pressure and a constantly moving stroke. Use overlapping multidirectional strokes on each tooth.

14. After completion of appointment, put on utility gloves. Flush the unit with distilled water for 30 seconds between patients. Remove barriers, clean, and use standard infection control procedures to disinfect the power unit.

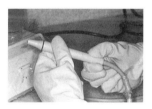

15. Uncouple the handpiece from the handpiece hose. Grip the larger, hard ribbed end of the handpiece hose, and pull straight out (do NOT twist).

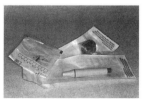

16. Sterilize the instrument tip, wrench, handpiece, and reservoir in autoclave or chemiclave. Do not immerse the handpiece in any liquids.

Instrument Tips

The variety of tip designs available for piezo units varies greatly from manufacturer to manufacturer. It is important to note that tips are not interchangeable from manufacturer to manufacturer (i.e., if you have an Amadent system, you must use Amadent tips.)

Recommended Use	EMS Tip Designs
• Anterior sextants, lingual aspect • Heavy calculus deposit • Supragingival use	 Lingual B
• Universal use • Moderate to heavy calculus removal • Supragingival use	 Universal A

continued

EMS Tip Designs	Recommended Use
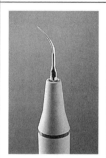 Perio Slim	• Universal use • Light calculus deposits and de-plaquing • Subgingival use in deep pockets
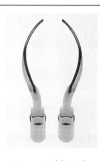 Interproximal Perio Pro	• Posterior sextants; two mirror-image tips with right and left configurations are needed to reach all surfaces • Root concavities and furcation areas • Light calculus deposits and de-plaquing • Subgingival use in deep pockets

continued

Recommended Use	EMS Tip Designs
• Posterior sextants; two mirror-image tips with right and left configurations are needed to reach all surfaces • Furcation areas and deplaquing of root surfaces • Light calculus deposits and de-plaquing • Subgingival use in deep pockets	 Balled-Furcation Perio Pro
• Universal use • Light calculus deposits • Subgingival use in deep pockets	 Round, Straight, Slim Tip

Section 4:

Sonic Instruments

At this time, most sonic units do not offer a wide selection of instrument tip designs. For this reason, many sonic mechanized instruments are limited to the removal of large- and moderately-sized calculus deposits.

SONIC INSTRUMENTS		
Examples	Dentsply/Midwest Quixonic KaVo Sonicflex Medidenta Micro-Motors	Scale-aire Scalerite Titan-S

Device	Conventional handpiece that attaches to dental
	    unit high-speed cable.
	Working tips screw directly onto handpiece with
	    the use of a special tool.	

Principle	This instrument is comprised of a handpiece containing a mechanical vibrating system and interchangeable screw-on scaling tips. Applying air pressure to the handpiece actuates the mechanical vibrating member that in turn causes the scaling tip to vibrate.	
Water	The primary purposes of water in the sonic systems are to cool the tip-tooth interface and flush the sulcus. Water flows through working tip; small diameter flow tube blocks easily and must be routinely cleaned with orthodontic wire.	

continued

Vibration	Sonic Vibration Frequency: Tip vibration is in the range of 3,000 to 8,000 cps (3–8 kHz). Sonic instruments are less efficient in removing calculus deposits than ultrasonic instruments because the sonic instrument tip vibrates at a slower rate; the slower rate of vibration is less vibrational action for calculus removal.
Tip	Sonic Tip Motion: Tips move typically in an orbital motion. Metal and plastic tips are available for some sonic handpieces; studies indicate that patients report more pain sensitivity to plastic than to metal sonic tips.

High magnification photography of the orbital tip movement of a sonic mechanized instrument. (Photograph courtesy of EMS Electro Medical Systems.)

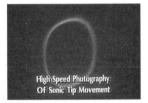

TECHNIQUE FOR USE

Example: The Midwest Quixonic Sonic Scaler

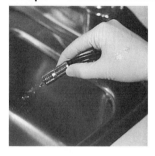

1. Position the dental unit water switch to the ON position. Hold the dental unit handpiece tubing over a sink. Step on the rheostat to activate a stream of running water. At the start of each day, run the water in this manner for 2 minutes. Between patients, run the water for 30 seconds. Turn the water unit OFF.

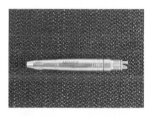

2. Obtain a sonic handpiece that has been sterilized in an autoclave or chemiclave.

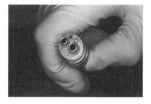

3. Connect the sonic handpiece to the handpiece tubing. The handpiece is easily attached to any 3- or 4-hold handpiece connector.

4. Select a sterilized instrument tip and
place the threaded
end into the hand-
piece. Hand tighten
the tip by turning it in
a clockwise direction
until fully sealed.

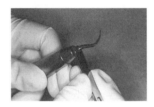

5. Use the wrench to
securely tighten the
tip. Do not use exces-
sive force with the
wrench. With the wa-
ter switch in the OFF
position, adjust the
air pressure to 40 to
50 pounds per square
inch (psi). Return wa-
ter switch to the ON
position. With the
handpiece operating
at 45 psi, slowly open
the dental unit's wa-
ter supply valve.
While holding the
handpiece over the
operatory sink, ad-
just the flow rate until
a fine mist ejects from
the tip.

6. Pre-procedural rinsing and irrigation. Ask the patient to rinse with an antimicrobial solution for 30
seconds. If appropriate, complete a preprocedural
subgingival irrigation of the treatment area before
instrumentation.

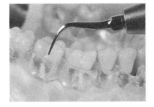

7. Establish an extra- or intraoral finger rest. Hold the tip off of the tooth surface as you step on the rheostat to activate the tip.

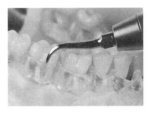

8. Adapt the instrument tip to the tooth surface. Position the tip so the length of the tip is adapted to the tooth surface in a manner similar to that of a calibrated periodontal probe.

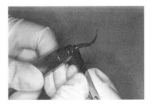

9. After completion of appointment, don utility gloves. To remove tip, turn tip counterclockwise with wrench to loosen.

10. Disconnect the sonic handpiece from the tubing. Scrub and rinse the external surface of the sonic handpiece under warm tap water. Dry thoroughly.

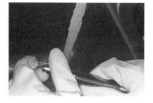

11. Place 3 drops of handpiece lubricant into the drive air tube. Reattach the handpiece to the tubing, and run for 15 seconds or until it reaches normal speed. Wipe off any excess lubricant with a dry gauze pad.

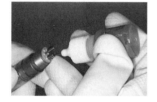

12. Place the sonic handpiece, tips, and wrench into autoclave pouches. Sterilize in autoclave or chemiclave.

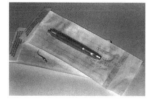

INSTRUMENT TIPS

The variety of tips available for sonic instruments tends to be more limited. Sonic tips usually are larger in size than the working ends of ultrasonic inserts and tips.

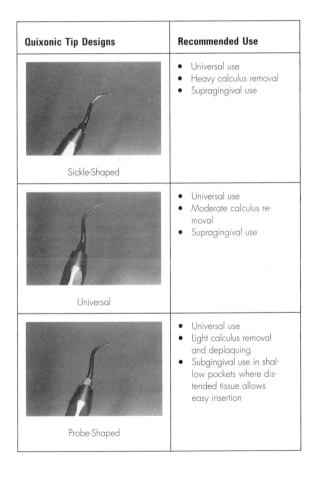

Quixonic Tip Designs	Recommended Use
Sickle-Shaped	• Universal use • Heavy calculus removal • Supragingival use
Universal	• Universal use • Moderate calculus removal • Supragingival use
Probe-Shaped	• Universal use • Light calculus removal and deplaquing • Subgingival use in shallow pockets where distended tissue allows easy insertion

SUMMARY SHEET: PROCEDURE FOR USE OF
MECHANIZED INSTRUMENTS

1. **Handpiece hose/dental unit tubing.** For ultrasonic units, run water through the handpiece hose a full 2 minutes at the start of the day and for 30 seconds between patients. For sonic instruments, run water through dental unit tubing for a full 2 minutes at start of the day and for 30 seconds between patients. Running the water in this manner flushes stagnant water from the hose or tubing.

2. **Tip selection.** Select the appropriate instrument tip for the task at hand. Use larger tips for removal of heavy calculus deposits and thin tips for light deposits, de-plaquing, and endotoxin removal.

3. **Power setting.** Adjust the power to the lowest setting at which a particular tip functions properly. The HIGH power setting should be avoided. Manual tuning of the power frequency is recommended when using thin instrument tips; these tips may damage the root surface if used on a high power setting.

4. **Water setting.** Adjust the water spray to create a light mist or halo effect at the instrument tip, with no excess dripping of water. Insufficient water flow over the tip can result in trauma to the pulp.

5. **Patient position.** Position patient in a normal supine position with the head turned to one side, toward or away from the clinician, depending on the area to be instrumented. This head position causes the water to pool in the cheek area of the mouth, which increases patient comfort and facilitates evacuation.

6. **Suction.** Provide high-volume suction with continual clearance for patient comfort and to prevent inhalation of contaminated water spray.

7. **Retraction.** Use fingers of the nondominant hand to hold the patient's lip or cheek in a cupped position away from the dental arch. The cupped tissues will tend to keep the water spray inside the mouth.

8. **Grasp.** Use a light, relaxed grasp.

9. **Instrument adaptation.** Adapt the side of the last several millimeters of the working end to the tooth surface. The working end is positioned in a manner similar to that of a periodontal probe with the length of the tip parallel to the long axis of the tooth. AVOID direct application of the tip of the working end ("point") to the tooth surface.

10. **Stroke pressure.** Apply light stroke pressure; heavy stroke pressure is unnecessary and can damage the tooth surface.

11. **Stroke pattern.** Use a brushlike motion. Overlapping multidirectional strokes are used to cover every square millimeter of the root surface.

12. **Stroke technique.** Keep the tip moving at all times. To remove heavier deposits, keep the tip in constant motion while making light strokes in a brushlike motion up and down over the area. It may take several minutes for heavy deposit removal.

Section 5:

References and Suggested Readings

Infection Control Issues: Aerosols, Pre-treatment Mouthrinses, Waterline Biofilms

Bentley, C.D., Burkhart, N.W., Crawford, J.J.: Evaluating spatter and aerosol contamination during dental procedures. J Am Dent Assoc May;125(5):579-84, 1994.

Christensen, R.P., Robison, R.A., Robinson, D.F., Ploeger, B.J., Leavitt, R.W.: Efficiency of 42 brands of face masks and 2 face shields in preventing inhalation of airborne debris. Gen Dent Nov-Dec; 39(6):414-21, 1991.

Dajani, A.S., Biano, A.L., Chung, K.G., et. al.: Prevention of bacterial endocarditis: recommendations of the American Heart Association. JAMA 264:2919-22, 1990.

Dental unit waterline contamination. Clin Res Assoc Newslet March;21(3), 1997.

Eleazer, P.D., Schuster, G.S., Weathers, D.R.: A chemical treatment regimen to reduce bacterial contamination in dental waterlines. J Am Dent Assoc May;128(5):617-23, 1997.

Fayle, S.A., Pollard, M.A.: Decontamination of dental unit water systems: a review of current recommendations. Br Dent J Nov 23;181(10):369-72, 1996.

Fine, D.H., Korik, I., Furgang, D., Myers, R., Olshan, A., Barnett, ML., Vincent, J.: Assessing pre-procedural subgingival irrigation and rinsing with an antiseptic mouthrinse to reduce bacteremia. J Am Dent Assoc May;127(5):641-2, 645-6, 1996.

Harrel, S.K.: Clinical use of an aerosol-reduction device with an ultrasonic scaler. Compend Contin Educ Dent Dec;17(12):1185-93; quiz 1194, 1996.

King, T.B., Muzzin, K.B., Berry, C.W., Anders, L.M.: The effectiveness of an aerosol reduction device for ultrasonic scalers. J Periodontol Jan;68(1):45-9, 1997.

Larato, D., Ruskin, P.F., Martin, A.: Effect of an ultrasonic scaler on bacterial counts in air. J Periodontol 38:550, 1967.

Logothetis, D.D., Martinez-Welles, J.M.: Reducing bacterial aerosol contamination with a chlorhexidine gluconate. J Am Dent Assoc Dec;126(12):1634-9, 1995.

Miller, C.H.: Infection control. Dent Clin North Am Apr;40(2):437-56, 1996.

Miller, C.H.: Microbes in dental unit water. J Calif Dent Assoc Jan;24(1):47-52, 1996.

Miller, R.L.: Characteristics of blood-containing aerosols generated by common powered dental instruments. Am Industr Hyg Assoc J Jul;56(7):670-6, 1995

Molinari, J.A.: Face masks: effective personal protection. Compend Contin Educ Dent Sep;17(9):818-21, 1996.

Molinari, J.A.: Waterborne microorganisms: colonization, contamination, and disease potential—Part 1. Compend Contin Educ Dent Oct;15(10):1192-6, 1994.

Molinari, J.A.: Waterborne microorganisms: questions about health-care problems and solutions—Part 2. Compend Contin Educ Dent Feb;16(2):130-2, 1995.

Peters, E., McGaw, W.T.: Dental unit water contamination. J Can Dent Assoc Jun;62(6):492-5, 1996.

Recommended infection-control practices for dentistry. MMWR Morb Mortal Wkly Rep 35:237, 1986.

Waggoner, M.B.: The new CDC surgical water recommendations: why they should be implemented and what they require. Compend Contin Educ Dent Jun;17(6):612-4, 616-20 passim; quiz 628, 1996.

Williams, J.F., Andrews, N., Santiago, J.I.: Microbial contamination of dental unit waterlines: current preventive measures and emerging options. Compend Contin Educ Dent Jul;17(7):691-4, 696-8 passim, quiz 709, 1996.

Williams, J.F., Molinari, J.A., Andrews, N.: Microbial contamination of dental unit waterlines: origins and characteristics. Compend Contin Educ Dent Jun;17(6):538-40, 542 passim, quiz 558, 1996.

Williams, H.N., Paszko-Kolva, C., Shahamat, M., Palmer, C., Pettis, C., Kelley J.: Molecular techniques reveal high prevalence of Legionella in dental units. J Am Dent Assoc Aug;127(8):1188-93, 1996.

Williams, H.N., Baer, M.L., Kelley, J.I.: Contribution of biofilm bacteria to the contamination of the dental unit water supply. J Am Dent Assoc Sep;126(9):1255-60, 1996.

Mechanized Instruments

Anderson, G.B., Plotzke, A.E., Morrison, E.C., Caffesse, R.G.: Effectiveness of an irrigating solution utilized during ultrasonic scaling. Quintessence Int Dec;26(12):849-58, 1995.

Baehni, P., Thilo, B., Chapuis, B., Pernet, D.: Effects of ultrasonic and sonic scalers on dental plaque microflora in vitro and in vivo. J Clin Periodontol Aug;19(7), 455-9, 1992.

Biagini, G., Checchi, L., Pelliccioni, G.A., Solmi, R.: In vitro growth of periodontal fibroblasts on treated cementum. Quintessence Int May;23(5):335-40, 1992.

Boretti, G., Zappa, U., Graf, H., Case, D.: Short-term effects of phase I therapy on crevicular cell populations. J Periodontol Mar;66(3), 235-40, 1995.

Bower, R.: Furcation morphology relative to periodontal treatment. Furcation entrance architecture. J Periodont 50:23, 1979.

Bray, K.K.: Reaching consensus on power-driven instrumentation: Proceedings from the 1996 World Workshop in Periodontics. Access Am Dent Hyg Assoc Jan;12 (1), 28-31, 1998.

Bray, K.K.: Innovations in periodontal debridement: Reexamining the role of power-driven scaling. Dent Hyg Connection 1(1):1-6, 1996.

Chapple, I.L., Walmsley, A.D., Saxby, M.S., Moscrop, H.: Effect of instrument power setting during ultrasonic scaling upon treatment outcome. J Periodontol Sept;66(9):756-60, 1995.

Chapple, I.L., Walmsley, A.D., Saxby, M.S., Moscrop, H.: Effect of subgingival irrigation with chlorhexidine during ultrasonic scaling. J Periodontol Oct;63(10):812-6, 1992.

Checchi, L., Pelliccioni, G.A.: Hand versus ultrasonic instrumentation in the removal of endotoxins from root surfaces in vitro. J Periodontol Jun;59(6):398-402, 1988.

Cavitron Ultrasonic Cleaning Tips with very fine, slim design. Clin Res Assoc Newslet Nov;1993.

Cobb, C.: Non-surgical pocket therapy: Mechanical debridement. (Proceedings of the 1996 World Workshop in Periodontology) Ann Periodontol 1(1), 1996.

Croft, L.K.: Ultrasonics in periodontal therapy—the paradigm has changed. Tex Dent J Apr;112(4):7, 9, 11-2, 1995.

Cross-Poline, G.N., Stach, D.J., Newman, S.M.: Effects of curet and ultrasonics on root surfaces. Am J Dent Jun;8(3):131-3, 1995.

DENTSPLY Cavitron: Instructional Manual DENTSPLY/Cavitron Prophy Jet C-300, Dental Prophylaxis Unit. York, PA: DENTSPLY International.

Dragoo, M.R., Wheeler, B.G.: Clinical evaluation of subgingival debridement with ultrasonic instruments used by trained and untrained operators. Gen Dent May-Jun;44(3):234-7, 1996.

Fine, D.H., Korik, I., Furgang, D., Myers, R., Olshan, A., Barnett, M.L., Vincent, J.: Assessing pre-procedural subgingival irrigation and rinsing with an antiseptic mouthrinse to reduce bacteremia. J Am Dent Assoc May 127(5):641-2, 645-6, 1996.

Fleischer, H., Mellonig, J.T., Brayer, W.K., Gray, J.L., Barnett, J.D.: Scaling and root planing efficacy in multirooted teeth. J Periodontol 60:402, 1989.

Fukazawa, E., Nishimura, K.: Superficial cemental curettage: its efficacy in promoting improved cellular attachment on human root surfaces previously damaged by periodontitis. J Periodontol Feb;65(2):168-76, 1994.

Hallmon, W.W., Waldrop, T.C., Meffert, R.M., Wade, B.W.: A comparative study of the effects of metallic, nonmetallic, and sonic instrumentation on titanium abutment surfaces. Int J Oral Maxillofac Implants Jan-Feb;11(1):96-100, 1996.

Hawkins, P.: Micro ultrasonics. Contemporary periodontal instrumentation. Access Am Dent Hyg Assoc July;10(6), 25-28, 1996.

Hermann, J.S., Rieder, C., Rateitschak, K.H., Hefti, A.F.: Sonic and ultrasonic scalers in a clinical comparison. A study in non-instructed patients with gingivitis or slight adult periodontitis. Schweiz Monatsschr Zahnmed 105(2):165-70, 1995.

Hou, G.L., Tsai, C.C., Weisgold, A.S.: Ultrasonic scaling therapy in advanced periodontitis. IV. A long-term study over six years. Kao Hsiung I Hsueh Ko Hsueh Tsa Chih Feb;13(2):103-16, 1997.

Hou, G.L., Tsai, C.C., Weisgold, A.S.: The effect of ultrasonic scaling therapy in periodontitis III. A longitudinal study over three years. Kao Hsiung I Hsueh Ko Hsueh Tsa Chih Jan;12(1):25-35, 1996.

King, T.B., Muzzin, K.B., Berry, C.W., Anders, L.M.: The effectiveness of an aerosol reduction device for ultrasonic scalers. J Periodontol Jan;68(1):45-9, 1997.

Kocher, T., Plagmann, H.C.: Heat propagation in dentin during instrumentation with different sonic scaler tips. Quintessence Int Apr;27(4):259-64, 1996.

Laird, W.R., Walmsley, A.D.: Ultrasound in dentistry. Part 1: Biophysical interactions. J Dent Feb;19(1):14-7, 1991.

Mankodi, S., Ross, N.M., Mostler, K: Clinical efficiency of Listerine in inhibiting and reducing plaque and experimental gingivitis. J Clin Periodontol 14:285, 1987.

McAllister, B., Narayanan, A.S., Miki, X., et al.: Isolation of a fibroblast attachment protein from cementum. J Periodont Res 25(2):99-105, 1990.

McInnes, C., Engel, D., Martin, R.W.: Fimbria damage and removal of adherent bacteria after exposure to acoustic energy. Oral Microbial Immunol Oct;8(5):277-82, 1993.

McInnes, C., Engel, D., Moncla, B.J., Martin, R.W.: Reduction in adherence of Actinomyces viscosus after exposure to low-frequency acoustic energy. Oral Microbiol Immunol Jun;7(3):171-6, 1992.

Moore, J., Wilson, M., Kieser, J.: The distribution of bacterial lipopolysaccharide (endotoxin) in relation to periodontally-involved root surfaces. J Clin Periodontol 13(8):748-51,1986.

Nakib, N.M., Bissada, N.F., Simmelink, J.W., Goldstine, S.N.: Endotoxin penetration into root cementum of periodontally involved teeth. J Periodontol 53:368, 1982.

Nosal, G., Scheidt, M., O'Neal, R., Van Dyke. T.: The penetration of lavage solution into the periodontal pocket during ultrasonic instrumentation. J Periodontol 62:554, 1991.

Nunn, P.J.: Sonic or ultrasonic?—Piezoelectric or magnetostrictive? Those are the questions! Access Am Dent Hyg Assoc Nov;10(9), 1996.

Nyman, S., Westfelt, E., Sarhed, G., Karring, T.: Role of "diseased" root cementum in healing following treatment of periodontal disease: A clinical study. J Clin Periodontol Aug;15(7):464-68, 1988.

O'Hehir, T.E.: Periodontal debridement therapy. Access Am Dent Hyg Assoc May-June;9:49, 1995.

Proceedings of the 1996 World Workshop in Periodontology: Non-surgical pocket therapy: Mechanical debridement. Ann Periodontol 1(1), 1996.

Räuhling, A., Kocher, T., Kreusch, J., Plagmann, H.C.: Treatment of subgingival implant surfaces with Teflon-coated sonic and ultrasonic scaler tips and various implant curettes. An in vitro study. Clin Oral Implants Res Mar;5(1):19-29, 1994.

Rosenberg, R.M., Ash, M.M.: The effect of root roughness on plaque accumulation and gingival inflammation. J Periodontol 45:146, 1974.

Shah, S., Walmsley, A.D., Chapple, I.L., Lumley, P.J.: Variability of sonic scaling tip movement. J Clin Periodontol Nov;21(10):705-9, 1994.

Smart, G.J., Wilson, M., Davies, E.H., Kieser, J.B.: The assessment of ultrasonic root surface debridement by determination of residual endotoxin levels. J Clin Periodontol Mar;17(3):174-8, 1990.

Suzuki, J.B., Delisle, A.L.: Pulmonary actinomycosis of periodontal origin. J Periodontol 55:581, 1984.

Torfason, T., Kiger, R., Selvig, K., et al: Clinical improvement of gingival conditions following ultrasonic versus hand instrumentation of periodontal pockets. J Clin Periodontol 6(3):165-76, 1979.

Walmsley, A.D., Walsh, T.F., Laird, W.R., Williams, A.R.: Effects of cavita-
    tional activity on the root surface of teeth during ultrasonic scaling.
    J Clin Periodontol May;17(5):306-12, 1990.
Walmsley, A.D.: Potential hazards of the dental ultrasonic descaler. Ultra-
    sound Med Biol 14:15, 1988.
Young, N.A.: Periodontal debridement: Re-examining non-surgical instrumen-
    tation. Part II: Expanding the role of ultrasonic and sonic instrumenta-
    tion. Semin Dent Hyg 5:1-7, 1995.

7

Fulcruming Techniques for the Experienced Clinician

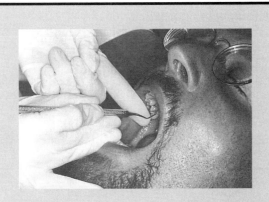

In this chapter

Section 1:

The Modified Pen Grasp

RIGHT-HANDED CLINICIAN

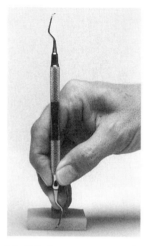 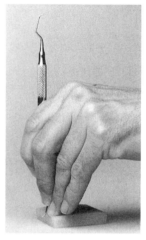

Modified pen grasp: side view, right-handed clinician

Modified pen grasp: front view, right-handed clinician

LEFT-HANDED CLINICIAN

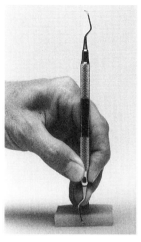 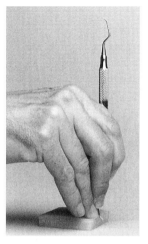

Modified pen grasp: side view, left-handed clinician

Modified pen grasp: front view, left-handed clinician

FINGER IDENTIFICATION

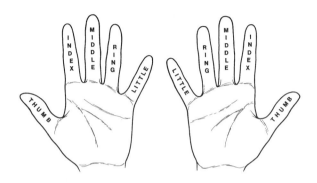

Basic Elements of the Instrument Grasp

Digit(s)	Location	Function
Index and Thumb	On the handle	Hold the instrument
Middle	Rests lightly on the shank	Helps to guide the working end Feels vibrations of working end
Ring	On oral structure—often on a tooth surface	Stabilizes hand for control and leverage
Little	Near ring finger in a natural relaxed manner	None

FINE TUNING

Apply the criteria described below to fine-tune your instrument grasp.

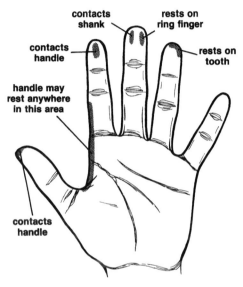

Right-Handed Operator

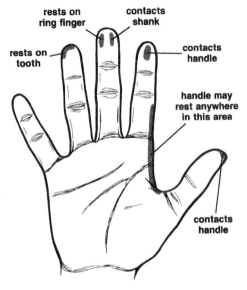

Left-Handed Operator

Section 2:

Standard Fulcruming Techniques

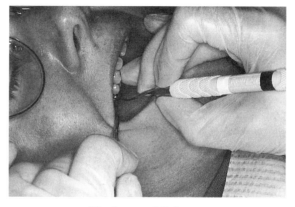

The Intraoral Fulcrum

THE INTRAORAL FULCRUM

Technique	Tip of the ring finger rests on a stable tooth surface
Location	On the same arch as the treatment area, near the tooth being instrumented
Advantages	• Provides the most stable, secure support for the clinician's hand • Provides leverage, strength, and stroke control during instrumentation • Provides excellent tactile information to the clinician's fingers during instrumentation • Allows the hand and instrument to work together effectively • Permits precise stroke control • Allows forceful stroke pressure with the least amount of stress to the clinician's hand and fingers • Decreases the likelihood of injury to the patient if he or she moves unexpectedly while the clinician is working
Disadvantage	• May be difficult to obtain parallelism for deep pocket access or when edentulous areas preclude the use of intraoral fulcrums

Section 3:

Alternative Fulcruming Techniques

Fulcruming techniques can be classified into two categories: (1) standard and (2) alternative. The standard fulcruming technique consists of using an intraoral fulcrum on a tooth surface as close as possible to the tooth being instrumented. Alternative fulcruming techniques include extraoral and advanced fulcrums.

Before attempting alternative fulcruming techniques, the clinician should have mastered the fundamentals of the neutral position and standard fulcruming technique. Bad habits with fundamental techniques cannot be corrected by the use of alternative fulcrums. A clinician with poor fundamental techniques will compound his or her problems by attempting to use alternative fulcrums. Unorthodox methods of instrumentation may serve as a quick fix for achieving an end-product but this is usually at the expense of the clinician's musculoskeletal system.

Alternative fulcruming techniques are not intended to replace the intraoral fulcrum. The basic intraoral fulcrum places the least amount of strain on the clinician's muscles. An intraoral finger rest, as close as possible to the area being instrumented, reduces the amount of force the clinician must exert in order to remove the calculus deposit. An alternative fulcrum should be used if an intraoral fulcrum is not effective or possible. Proper use of alternative fulcrums in combination with correct fundamental techniques can serve as a useful method for achieving parallelism for deep pocket access and it is also advantageous when edentulous areas preclude the use of intraoral fulcrums.

Fulcruming Techniques

Categories	Types	Effectiveness
Standard Fulcruming Technique	1. Intraoral Fulcrum	Highly effective
Alternative Fulcruming Techniques	1. Basic Extraoral Fulcrums	Least effective
	2. Advanced Fulcrums • Modified Intraoral • Piggy-Backed Intraoral • Cross-Arch • Opposite Arch • Finger-on-Finger • Stabilized	Very Effective

ADVANTAGES AND DISADVANTAGES

Alternative fulcruming techniques should be used selectively (1) in areas of limited access and (2) in order to maintain neutral body position.

ADVANTAGES OF ALTERNATIVE FULCRUMING TECHNIQUES

1. Work well in areas of limited access such as, maxillary second and third molars
2. Allow for improved parallelism of the lower instrument shank to the tooth surface
3. Permit easier access to deep pockets, especially for access to the base of pockets more than 4 mm in depth on maxillary posterior teeth
4. In some cases, make it easier for the clinician to maintain the wrist in neutral position

DISADVANTAGES OF ALTERNATIVE FULCRUMING TECHNIQUES

1. Require more muscle coordination and instrumentation skill by the clinician
2. With stabilized fulcrums, the clinician is unable to use indirect vision with a mirror.
3. With finger-on-finger fulcrums, the supporting finger could sustain an instrument stick if the clinician slips.
4. Some of the alternative fulcruming techniques, require the clinician to grasp the instrument lower on the handle; this grasp position usually makes it impossible to maintain the middle finger on the shank of the instrument. When the middle finger is NOT resting on the shank: (1) tactile information to the fingers is greatly reduced, and (2) stroke control and pressure are greatly reduced.
5. Some alternative techniques can cause additional stress to the clinician's hand and fingers during instrumentation.
6. Some alternative fulcruming techniques are not well tolerated by patient's with limited opening or TMJ problems.

OBTAINING PARALLELISM FOR DEEP POCKET ACCESS

When working within a deep pocket, sometimes it is difficult to obtain parallelism of the lower shank with the root surface to be treated. This is especially true for the maxillary molars. Alternative fulcruming techniques are useful in obtaining parallelism.

Using an **intraoral fulcrum,** it is sometimes difficult to obtain access to the proximal surfaces of maxillary posterior teeth.

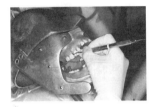

This close-up photograph shows the clinician having difficulty attaining parallelism of the lower shank to the mesial surface of the maxillary molar when using an **intraoral fulcrum.**

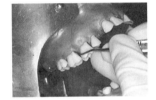

An **extraoral fulcrum on the opposite arch:** The extraoral fulcrum makes it easier for the clinician to obtain parallelism of the lower shank to the proximal surfaces of maxillary molars.

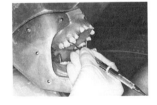

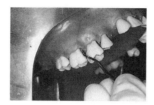

Extraoral fulcrum permits improved parallelism to obtain access to pocket more than 4 mm in depth.

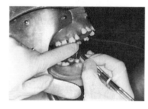

A **stabilized fulcrum** allows the clinician to establish parallelism. An additional advantage is placing a finger from the non-dominant hand against the shank to concentrate lateral pressure backward against the mesial surface.

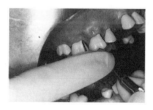

The **stabilized fulcrum** increases stroke control and pressure when using an extraoral or opposite arch fulcrum.

TYPES OF ALTERNATIVE FULCRUMING TECHNIQUES
Basic Extraoral Fulcrums

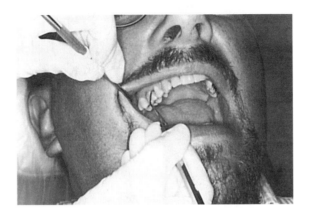

The **basic extraoral fulcrum** involves resting the fingers or palm of the hand against the patient's chin or cheeks.

ADVANTAGES OF THE BASIC EXTRAORAL FULCRUM

1. Provides greater parallelism for access to the base of pockets more than 4 mm in depth on maxillary posterior teeth, especially the distals of the second and third molars.
2. Provides neutral wrist positioning and allows the hand/arm to function as a unit.

DISADVANTAGES OF THE BASIC EXTRAORAL FULCRUM

1. Usually requires the clinician to grasp the instrument lower on the handle, reducing stroke control and tactile information to the fingers.
2. Causes greatest stress to the clinician's hand and fingers.
3. Least effective of all fulcruming techniques; the technique of last resort.

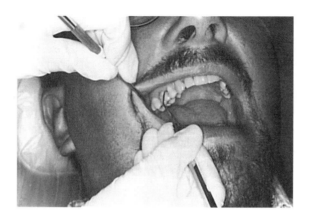

Folded knuckle technique establishes an extraoral fulcrum by folding your knuckles against the patient's chin.

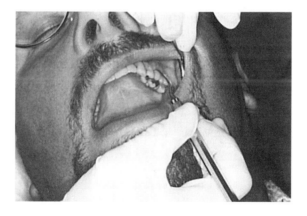

Chin cup technique is an equally effective extraoral fulcrum established by cupping the patient's chin with the palm of your hand.

Modified Intraoral Fulcrum

The modified intraoral fulcrum is a variation of the modified pen grasp and an intraoral fulcrum. In the standard modified pen grasp, the terminal phalanx of the middle finger is in contact with the ring finger. In the modified intraoral fulcrum, the proximal phalanx of the middle finger is in contact with the ring finger.

The modified intraoral fulcrum should not be confused with a split fulcrum. In a split fulcrum, there is no contact between the middle and ring fingers. The fingers cannot function as a unit with split fulcrum; over time, this technique may result in a musculoskeletal injury.

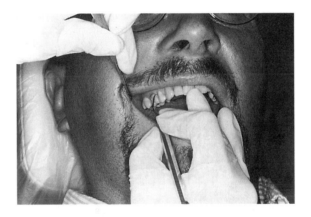

The **modified intraoral fulcrum** alters the point of contact between the middle and ring fingers. Here, the fulcrum finger rests on the maxillary anterior tooth while the treatment area is a posterior tooth. There is contact between the middle finger and the ring finger in the area of the proximal phalanx.

ADVANTAGES OF THE MODIFIED INTRAORAL FULCRUM

Advantages include all of the advantages of the modified pen grasp and basic fulcrum:
1. Provides good tactile sensitivity during instrumentation
2. Provides stability and control during instrumentation
3. Provides a stable, secure support for the clinician's hand
4. Decreases the likelihood of injury to the patient and the clinician if the patient moves unexpectedly during instrumentation
5. Provides leverage, strength, and stroke control during instrumentation
6. Allows for positioning of the instrument in line with the long axis of the tooth
7. Improves access and parallelism

DISADVANTAGES OF THE MODIFIED INTRAORAL FULCRUM

This technique requires more muscle control and coordination than the modified pen grasp and basic fulcrum.

Piggy-Backed Intraoral Fulcrum

This fulcrum is accomplished by stacking the middle finger on the fulcrum finger in a piggy-back style.

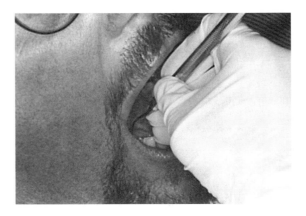

The **piggy-backed intraoral fulcrum** elevates the index finger and thumb by stacking the middle finger on top of the ring finger.

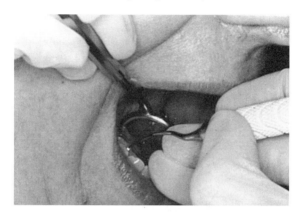

Piggy-backed intraoral fulcrum is helpful in gaining access to the lingual aspect of the mandibular molars.

ADVANTAGES OF THE PIGGY-BACKED INTRAORAL FULCRUM

1. Provides improved access to the lingual aspect of the mandibular molars
2. Aligns the fingers in close approximation
   - Providing improved transfer of the work of the stroke production onto the fulcrum finger
   - Enhancing the whole hand functioning as a unit from the wrist, eliminating digital (finger) activation

DISADVANTAGE OF THE PIGGY-BACKED INTRAORAL FULCRUM

Patients with small mouths cannot accommodate this fulcrum when the clinician has a large, broad hand size.

Cross-Arch Fulcrum

The cross-arch fulcrum is accomplished by establishing a finger rest on a tooth on the opposite side of the arch from the one being instrumented (e.g., establishing a finger rest on the left side of the mandible to instrument a mandibular right molar).

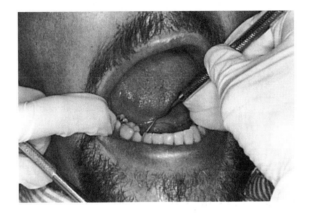

A **cross-arch fulcrum** is established on the opposite side of the arch from the treatment area; this fulcrum is most often used to gain access to the mandibular molars.

ADVANTAGE OF THE CROSS-ARCH FULCRUM

This technique allows improved access to the distals of the mandibular molars.

DISADVANTAGES OF THE CROSS-ARCH FULCRUM

1. Usually requires the clinician to grasp the instrument lower on the handle, reducing stroke control and tactile information to the fingers
2. Makes it more difficult to apply firm stroke pressure

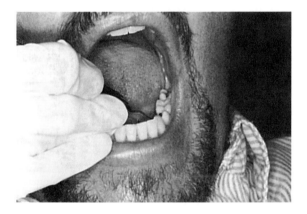

A **cross-arch fulcrum** on the mandibular right anteriors is used while working on the mandibular left premolars, lingual aspect.

Opposite Arch Fulcrum

The opposite arch fulcrum is an advanced fulcrum used to improve access and parallelism during instrumentation. Because it is an intraoral fulcrum, it is not as useful as the extraoral fulcrum on patients with limited opening. It has all the same advantages and disadvantages of the extraoral fulcrum.

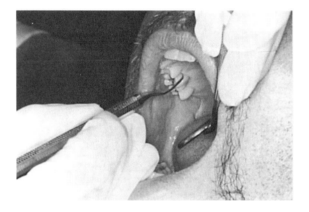

The **opposite arch fulcrum** is established on the opposite arch from the treatment area; in this example, the fulcrum is on the mandibular anterior teeth while working on the maxillary right first molar, lingual aspect.

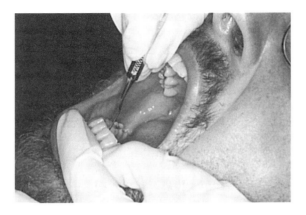

Here an **opposite arch fulcrum** on the maxillary anteriors is used to gain access to the lingual aspect of the mandibular anterior teeth.

ADVANTAGES OF THE OPPOSITE ARCH FULCRUM

1. Provides greater parallelism for access to the base of pockets more than 4 mm in depth, especially on maxillary posterior teeth
2. Provides neutral wrist positioning and allows the hand and arm to function as a unit

DISADVANTAGES OF THE OPPOSITE ARCH FULCRUM

1. Requires the clinician to grasp the instrument lower on the handle, reducing stroke control and tactile information to the fingers
2. Causes greater stress to the clinician's hand and fingers
3. The opposite arch fulcrum may be uncomfortable for patients with TMJ problems. The pressure of the fulcrum on the mandibular teeth places a strain on the muscles associated with TMJ disorders. For some patients this fulcrum can cause spasm and TMJ pain.

Finger-on-Finger Fulcrum

This type of fulcrum uses the index finger of the non-dominant hand by placing it on the occlusal surfaces of the teeth in the working area. The clinician can fulcrum in line with the long axis of the tooth to improve access and parallelism in instrumentation.

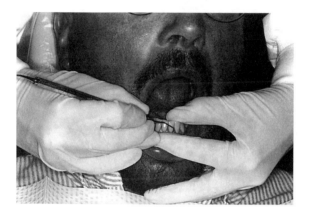

In the **finger-on-finger fulcrum,** a finger of the non-dominant hand serves as the resting point for the fulcrum finger of the dominant hand. In this example, a right-handed operator is seated behind the patient. The index finger of the clinician's left hand serves as a resting point for the right hand while instrumenting the mandibular anteriors. Fingers of the non-dominant hand are used for retraction of the lip, and the thumb can be used to control the patient's tongue, if necessary.

ADVANTAGES OF THE FINGER-ON-FINGER FULCRUM

1. Improved parallelism
2. Greater access to deep pockets

DISADVANTAGES OF THE FINGER-ON-FINGER FULCRUM

1. Possibility of an instrument stick to the finger of the non-dominant hand if the clinician slips
2. Cannot use the non-dominant hand for retraction or indirect vision

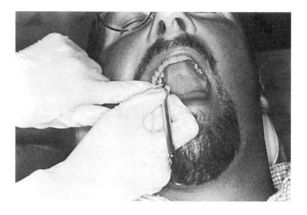

Finger-on-finger fulcrum demonstrated by a right-handed clinician for the maxillary right molars, lingual aspect. The clinician's right fulcrum finger is resting on the index finger of the left hand.

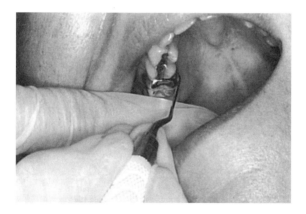

A close-up view of a **finger-on-finger fulcrum** used by a right-handed clinician while instrumenting the maxillary right posteriors, lingual aspect. The fulcrum finger of the right hand rests on the index finger of the left hand.

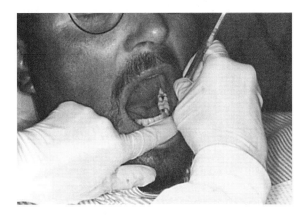

Finger-on-finger fulcrum demonstrated by a right-handed clinician for the mandibular left posteriors, facial aspect. The clinician's right ring finger is resting on the index finger of the left hand.

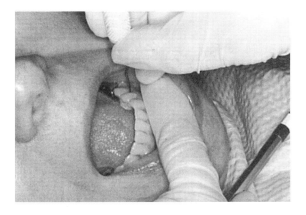

A close-up view of a **finger-on-finger fulcrum** used by a right-handed clinician while instrumenting the mandibular left posteriors, facial aspect. The fulcrum finger of the right hand rests on the index finger of the left hand.

Stabilized Fulcrum

This fulcrum also is known as a reinforced or supplemental fulcrum. A **stabilized fulcrum** is accomplished by using the thumb or index finger of the non-dominant hand (i.e., mirror hand). The thumb or index finger of the non-dominant hand is placed on the shank of the instrument to (1) direct lateral pressure with the cutting edge against the tooth and (2) help control the tip of the instrument. The stabilized fulcrum may be used with either an intraoral or an extraoral fulcrum.

For a **stabilized fulcrum,** a finger of the non-dominant hand applies pressure against the instrument shank to concentrate stroke pressure against the tooth surface being instrumented.

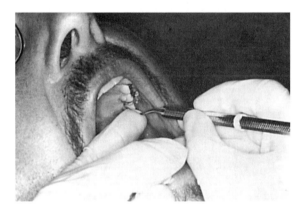

In this example demonstrated by a right-handed clinician, the index finger of the left hand is placed behind the shank to press the cutting edge forward against the distal surface of the molar. This technique is especially useful in an area where the calculus is tenacious and the tissue is fragile.

ADVANTAGES OF THE STABILIZED FULCRUM

1. Provides added support for the removal of tenacious subgingival calculus
2. Reduces the muscle strain and workload for the dominant hand, resulting in less fatigue for the clinician; less likelihood of musculoskeletal injury to the fingers of the dominant hand
3. Provides added control and stability for the clinician who is learning an extraoral fulcrum and, therefore, facilitates the transition from an intraoral to an extraoral fulcruming technique

DISADVANTAGE OF THE STABILIZED FULCRUM

Cannot be used with indirect vision because the non-dominant hand is used to stabilize the fulcrum and is not available to hold the dental mirror for retraction or indirect vision

A **stabilized fulcrum** demonstrated by a right-handed clinician for the maxillary right posteriors, lingual aspect. The clinician is instrumenting the mesial surface of the first molar. The clinician is using an opposite arch fulcrum and using the index finger of the left hand to stabilize the working end.

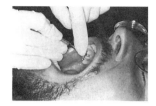

A close-up view of the **stabilized fulcrum** shown in the photograph above. The right-handed clinician is using the index finger of the left hand to press against the front side of the shank to concentrate lateral pressure back against the mesial surface of the first molar.

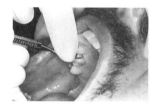

A **stabilized fulcrum** demonstrated by a right-handed clinician for the maxillary right posteriors, lingual aspect. In this example, the clinician is instrumenting the distal surface of the first molar.

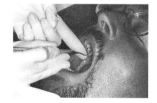

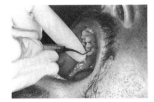

A close-up view of the **stabilized fulcrum** shown in the photograph above. The right-handed clinician positions the index finger of the left hand behind the shank to concentrate lateral pressure forward against the distal surface of the first molar.

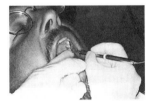

A **stabilized fulcrum** demonstrated by a right-handed clinician for the maxillary left posteriors, lingual aspect. In this example, the clinician is instrumenting the distal surface of the first molar. The clinician is using an opposite arch fulcrum on the mandibular arch.

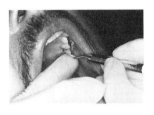

A close-up view of the **stabilized fulcrum** shown in the photograph above. The right-handed clinician positions the index finger of the left hand behind the shank to concentrate lateral pressure forward against the distal surface of the first molar.

A **stabilized fulcrum** demonstrated by a right-handed clinician while instrumenting the facial surfaces of the mandibular anterior teeth. The clinician is seated behind the patient and using an intraoral fulcrum. The thumb of the left hand is used to retract the lip.

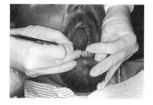

A close-up view of the **stabilized fulcrum** shown in the photograph above. The right-handed clinician positions the index finger of the left hand on the shank to stabilize a circumferential instrument stroke. The stabilized fulcrum helps to control the horizontal stroke by concentrating the lateral pressure specifically on the cutting edge.

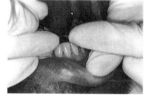

8

Sharpening Hand-Activated Instruments

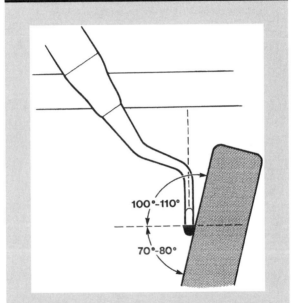

100°-110°

70°-80°

In this chapter

- Skill Practice: Establishing Correct Angulation
- Positioning Curets and Sickle Scalers for Sharpening

Section 2:

Equipment for Instrument Sharpening

- Sharpening Stones
- Equipment
- Work Area
- Sharpening Aid

Section 3:

Technique for Sharpening

- A Step-By-Step Guide
- Sharpening Periodontal Files

Section 4:

Sharpening Aids

- Sharpening Guide
- Directions for Use of Sharpening Guide

Section 5:

References and Suggested Readings

Section 1:

Introduction to Sharpening Concepts

ADVANTAGES OF USING A SHARP INSTRUMENT

The cutting edge or edges of hand-activated instruments must be sharp to achieve efficient and effective periodontal debridement with minimal tissue trauma. A sharp cutting edge allows:

Improved tactile sensitivity
A sharp cutting edge "grabs the tooth surface," making it easier to detect calculus deposits. A dull cutting edge will "roll over" the tooth surface, making it difficult to detect calculus deposits. It is difficult to remove calculus deposits if you cannot detect them.

Easier calculus removal
A sharp cutting edge "bites into" the calculus deposit, removing it in an efficient manner. A dull cutting edge will slide over the calculus deposit; it takes many more strokes to remove a deposit with a dull instrument. Dull cuttings edges often will burnish the calculus deposit, making it difficult to remove the calculus at all.

Improved stroke control
When making a calculus removal stroke, the clinician applies lateral pressure against the tooth and makes a scraping stroke in an apical direction. It is difficult to obtain lateral pressure with a dull cutting edge. As a result, it must be pressed with greater force against the tooth surface. This excessive force places strain on the clinician's musculoskeletal system. The greater force employed when using a dull cutting edge increases the likelihood of losing control of the instrument stroke. The clinician is more likely to slip and cut the tissue or obtain an instrument stick.

Reduced number of strokes
It takes fewer strokes to remove a calculus deposit with a
sharp cutting edge. Sharp instruments reduce the overall
treatment time.

Increased patient comfort
A sharp instrument allows the clinician to use less force
and make fewer, better controlled instrument strokes.
A sharp cutting edge, therefore, increases patient comfort and confidence in the treatment process.

Reduced clinician fatigue
A sharp cutting edge makes instrumentation more effective and efficient. A well-sharpened instrument reduces
stress to the clinician's fingers, hand, and wrist. A dull
cutting edge increases the likelihood of musculoskeletal injury.

UNDERSTANDING THE DESIGN FEATURES OF CURETS AND SICKLE SCALERS

To sharpen a hand-activated periodontal instrument correctly, you need to have a clear understanding of the
following design features of the working end: (1) the
cutting edge and (2) the relationship of the lateral surface
to the instrument face.

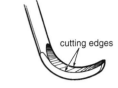

The cutting edge is formed by the union of the face and a lateral side. This illustration shows the two cutting edges of a universal curet. A sharp cutting edges is a **line.** It has length but no width.

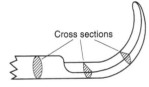

Cross sections

In order to understand **the relationship of the lateral surface to the instrument face,** you must view the working end in cross sections. The illustration shows a universal curet.

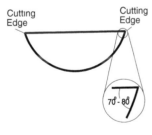

Cutting Edge

Cutting Edge

70° - 80°

The lateral surfaces meet the instrument face at an internal angle between 70° and 80°.

This 70° to 80° angulation is found on all:
(1) universal curets,
(2) area-specific curets, and
(3) sickle scalers.

A Dull Cutting Edge

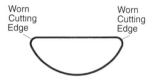

As the cutting edge is used against the tooth surface, the metal is gradually worn away creating **a dull cutting edge.** The cutting edge changes from a sharp point to a rounded, surface.

When the cutting edge is dull, the face and lateral surface meet in a wide, rounded surface. This rounded surface will slide over the calculus deposit instead of biting into it.

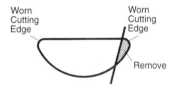

The shaded area on the illustration above shows the portion of the lateral surface that must be removed in **order to restore a fine, sharp cutting edge.**

To restore the original design of the working end, the lateral surface is ground away until it once again meets the instrument face at an internal angle between 70° to 80°.

Remember, this 70° to 80° angle is the same for all curets and sickle scalers.

SKILL PRACTICE: ESTABLISHING CORRECT ANGULATION

Follow the directions on this page to gain experience in establishing the correct angulation between the sharpening stone and the instrument face. Equipment for this practice session: (1) a rectangular sharpening stone and (2) the illustration on page 367.

Establish a 90° angle to the face.

1. Place your sharpening stone on the dotted line labeled as a 90° angle. Your sharpening stone is now positioned at a 90° angle to the instrument face. This position gives you a visual starting point from which to establish the correct angle between the sharpening stone and the instrument face.

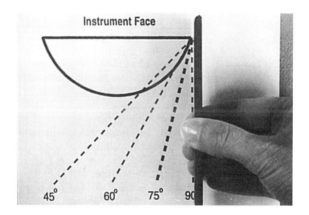

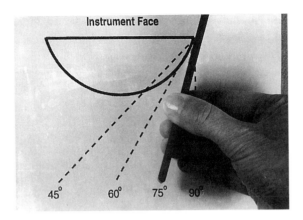

Correct angulation:

2.   Once again, begin by positioning the stone at a 90°
     angle to the face.

3.   Next, swing the lower end of the sharpening stone
     toward the instrument back. Align your stone with
     the dotted line labeled as a 75° angle.

4.   Your sharpening stone is now at the proper angle to
     the face. If you maintain this angle while sharpening,
     you will create a correctly recontoured cutting edge.
     You did not have to swing the lower end of the
     sharpening stone far to achieve the 75° angle.

Practice With Angles

Use this illustration to practice establishing the correct angle between the instrument face and your instrument stone.

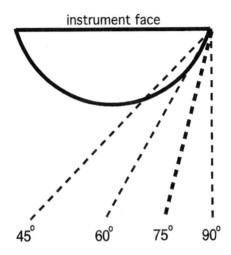

POSITIONING CURETS AND SICKLE SCALERS
FOR SHARPENING

> **Principle:** Position the working end so that the **face is parallel (=)** to the counter top.

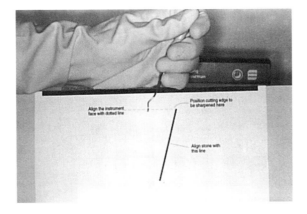

- Rest your nondominant hand on a stable counter or table. Grasp the instrument handle in the palm of your hand.

- Hold the instrument so that you are looking at the toe of the working end.

- Position the instrument handle so that the instrument face is parallel (=) to the counter top.

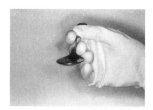

A spoonful of cough syrup. Imagine that the working end of your instrument is a tablespoon filled with red, sticky cough syrup. You must hold the spoon so that the sides of the bowl are level with each other or the cough syrup will spill!

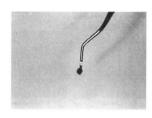

Imagine a curet face that is covered with red cough syrup. You must position the face so that it is level or the imaginary cough syrup will spill. This level position, with the instrument face parallel to the counter top, is the correct one for instrument sharpening.

Positioning a Universal Curet or a Sickle Scaler

Position the instrument face so that it is parallel (=) to the counter top.

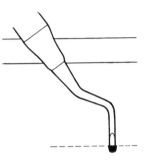

With a sickle or universal curet, when the face is positioned correctly, the lower shank will be perpendicular (⊥) to the counter top. Two cutting edges are sharpened on the working end of a sickle scaler or a universal curet.

Positioning an Area-Specific Curet

Position the instrument face so that it is parallel (=) to the counter top.

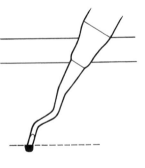

With an area-specific curet, when the face is positioned correctly, the lower shank will not be perpendicular to the counter top. One cutting edge, the lower cutting edge, is sharpened on the working end of an area-specific curet.

Equipment for
Instrument Sharpening

TYPES OF SHARPENING STONES

Type	Abrasive Texture	Use	Lubrication
Composition sharpening stone	Coarse	A synthetic (i.e., man-made) stone used for extensive reshaping of working ends that have been improperly sharpened or that have extremely dull, worn cutting edges. Use only on metal instruments.	Water
India stone	Medium	A synthetic stone used to sharpen dull cutting edges. Use only on metal instruments.	Water or oil
Arkansas stone	Fine	A natural stone used for routine sharpening of instruments. Use only on metal instruments.	Mineral oil
Ceramic stone	Fine	A synthetic stone used for routine sharpening of instruments. Use on metal instruments and certain plastic implant instruments; follow manufacturer's instructions for plastic instruments.	Water

SHARPENING STONES

Lubrication

During the sharpening process, particles of metal are removed from the surface of the working end. These metal shavings can become imbedded in the surface of the sharpening stone. The sharpening stone may be used in a dry state or it may be lubricated. Lubricating the sharpening stone with either water or oil will help to prevent the metal shavings from sticking to the surface of the stone. In addition, lubrication reduces frictional heat between the metal instrument and the stone. Stones that are used without lubrication will need to be replaced more frequently than stones used with lubricant.

The surface of the stone should be wiped with water or covered with a light coating of oil. One or two drops of oil is sufficient to lubricate the stone. A sharpening stone that can be lubricated with water is recommended for use when sharpening instruments during treatment at chairside. Distilled water can be used for sharpening during treatment.

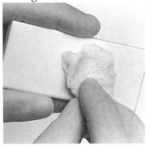

If you choose to lubricate your stone, lubricate it with distilled water or a few drops of oil.

When to Sharpen

Calculus removal will be easier and instruments will last longer if you sharpen the instruments after each use. Instruments on your instrument tray that were not used do not need to be sharpened; modern stainless steel instruments are not dulled by autoclaving. All instruments used during the appointment for debridement should be sharpened.

If you sharpen your instruments routinely after use, a few light strokes with the stone will restore a sharp cutting edge. Sharpening can be a quick, easy procedure if done in this manner.

Sharpening becomes a difficult and time-consuming process if instruments become dull through repeated use without sharpening. In this case, you will need to use many strokes with the stone to restore the cutting edge. Dull, neglected cutting edges require extensive recontouring. The original design features of the working end can be easily altered when extensive sharpening is necessary.

Care of Sharpening Stones

After using, wipe the surface of the stone with a wet 4 x 4 gauze square. Scrub the stone with a brush or clean ultrasonically. Dry stone on a paper towel; place in autoclave bag and sterilize.

EQUIPMENT

1. Clinicians need a heat-sterilized rectangular sharpening stone and/or a heat-sterilized tanged file for sharpening periodontal files. Refer to the section on sharpening periodontal files, later in this chapter, for more information.
2. Clinicians need a heat-sterilized plastic sharpening test stick to test the sharpness of the cutting edge.
3. Clinicians need protective eyewear. When sharpening non-sterile instruments during or after treatment, wear a mask and gloves, in addition, to protective eyewear.

WORK AREA

1. A stable work surface is essential for good sharpening technique. The countertop in the treatment room makes a good surface. The work area should be disinfected and covered with a barrier such as plastic wrap. The barrier should cover the top and side of the counter top.

2. A good light source, such as the dental unit light, should be directed over the working area.

3. A lighted magnifying lens is also helpful for examining the working end during sharpening.

SHARPENING AID

If you have difficulty maintaining the correct angulation of the sharpening stone to the instrument face, you may want to invest in a sharpening system. One excellent system is the PRU-DENT Sharpening System. This system consists of a sharpener base that holds the stone at the correct angulation for sharpening. The sharpener base is completely autoclavable. For information, contact PRU-DENT Dental Instrument Mfg., Co., at (312) 631-2339.

The PRU-DENT sharpening base holds a rectangular sharpening stone at the correct angle for instrument sharpening. This sharpening system will accommodate rectangular composition, Arkansas, and ceramic stones.

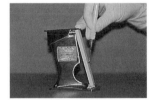

Section 3:

Technique for Sharpening

A STEP-BY-STEP GUIDE

Sharpening Sickle Scalers and Universal and Area-Specific Curets

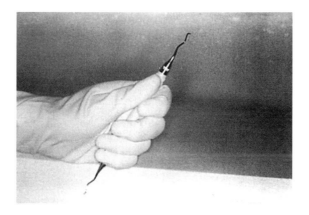

1. **Set-up work area and grasp instrument.**
Lubricate the sharpening stone.

Your <u>nondominant hand</u> is used to hold the instrument. Rest your hand and arm on the countertop. Grasp the instrument handle in the palm of your hand. Hold the length of the handle in a firm grasp. Stabilize the upper shank with your thumb.

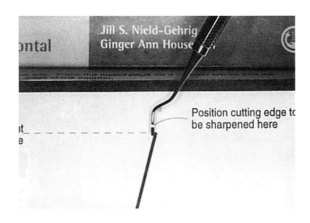

Position cutting edge to
be sharpened here

2. **Position the face. <u>For Sickle Scalers and Universal Curets:</u>**

<u>Right-Handed Clinician</u>
Point the tip or toe of the working end <u>toward</u> you to sharpen the right cutting edge.
Point the tip or toe of the working end away from you to sharpen the <u>other</u> cutting edge.

<u>Left-Handed Clinician</u>
Point the tip or toe of the working end <u>toward</u> you to sharpen the left cutting edge.
Point the tip or toe of the working end <u>away</u> from you to sharpen the <u>other</u> cutting edge.

   The photograph shows a universal curet with the toe pointing toward you.

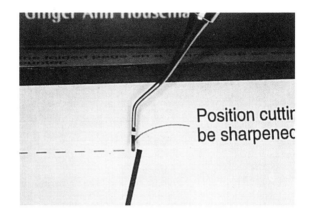

3. **Position the face. <u>For Area-Specific Curets:</u>**

<u>Right-Handed Clinician</u>
For all <u>ODD</u>-numbered working ends, point the toe <u>toward</u> you.
For all <u>EVEN</u>-numbered working ends, point the toe <u>away</u> from you.

<u>Left-Handed Clinician</u>
For all <u>EVEN</u>-numbered working ends, point the toe <u>toward</u> you.
For all <u>ODD</u>-numbered working ends, point the toe <u>away</u> from you.

The photograph shows a Gracey 13 in position for a right-handed clinician.

4. **Grasp the sharpening stone** in your dominant hand. Confine your grasp to the lower third of the stone. Grasp the stone on the edges so that your fingers do not get in the way when sharpening.

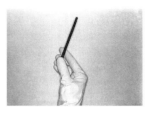

The photograph shows a right-handed clinician.

5. **Position the stone.**

Make sure that the instrument face is parallel to counter top. Imagine the face is covered with red cough syrup.

Position the stone perpendicular (⊥) to the instrument face. This position gives you a visual guideline for establishing the angulation.

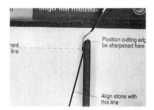

The photograph shows a right-handed clinician.

You only need to swing the lower portion of the stone slightly closer to the back of the instrument in order to establish the correct angle for sharpening.

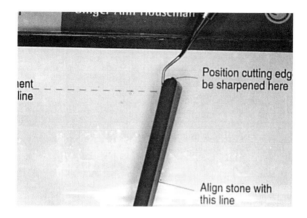

6. **Establish an angle of approximately 75°** for sharpening by swinging the lower part of the stone closer to the lateral surface and back of the instrument. If the stone is in the proper position, the lower part of the stone will tilt away from the palm of your dominant hand.

TECHNIQUE STRATEGY: SHARPEN THE CUTTING EDGE IN SECTIONS.

To maintain the original contour of the lateral surface, divide the cutting into 3 imaginary sections for sharpening.

Sharpen the imaginary sections, one by one, until you reach the toe (or tip) of the working end.

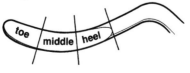

7. **Adapt the stone to the heel-third of the working end.** The photograph shows a bird's-eye-view looking down at the instrument face. Only the heel-third of the cutting edge is in contact with the surface of the sharpening stone.

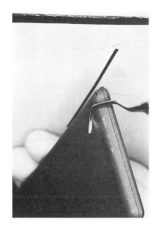

8. **Activate sharpening strokes.** Move the sharpening stone up and down in short, rhythmic strokes to remove metal from the lateral surface. If you sharpen an instrument after each use, you will need only a few, light strokes on the heel-third of the cutting edge. Finish each series of strokes in a down stroke to avoid leaving metal burs on the cutting edge.

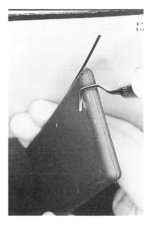

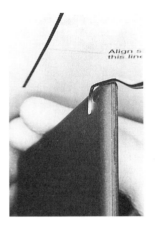

9. When the heel section is sharp, reposition the stone so that it is in contact with the middle-third of the cutting edge. Use a few up and down strokes to **sharpen the middle-third of the cutting edge.** End the strokes with a down stroke.

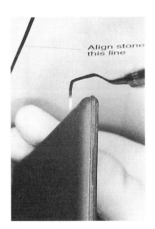

10. Reposition the stone so that it is in contact with the toe-third (or tip-third) of the cutting edge. **Sharpen the toe-third of the cutting edge.**

If sharpening a sickle scaler, skip to Step 13.

*If sharpening a curet, read ''Technique Strategy'' and pro-
ceed to Step 11.*

TECHNIQUE STRATEGY: RECONTOUR THE TOE OF A CURET.

When sharpening a curet, it is necessary to sharpen the toe in order
to maintain its rounded contour.

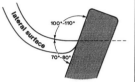

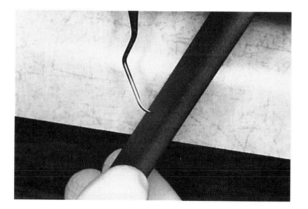

11. To recontour the curet toe, turn the working end
    so that you are looking at the lateral surface of the
    cutting edge. Be careful to keep the face parallel
    (=) to the counter top. Move the stone in up and
    down strokes as you work your way around the
    toe of the working end.

TECHNIQUE STRATEGY: RECONTOUR THE BACK OF A CURET.

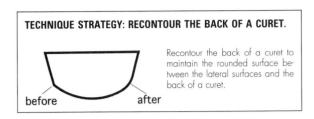

before   after

Recontour the back of a curet to maintain the rounded surface between the lateral surfaces and the back of a curet.

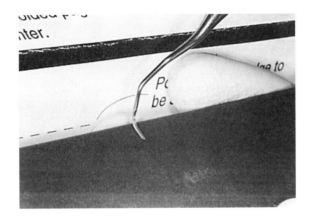

12. For curets, turn the working end so that you are looking at the toe. Use semicircular strokes to round the back of the curet.

13. **Grasp the plastic test stick.** Obtain a plastic test stick. Hold the stick at waist level in your non-dominant hand.

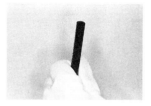

14. **Establish a finger rest on the top of the stick.** Hold the test stick so that you are looking down at the top of the stick. Establish a finger rest with the ring finger of your dominant hand on the top of the stick.

The photograph shows a right-handed clinician.

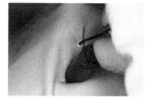

15. **Adapt the cutting edge.** Imagine that the stick is the crown of a molar tooth. The top of the stick is the occlusal surface; the sides of the stick are the facial, lingual, and proximal surfaces of the molar.

Position the stick so that you are looking down on the top. Adapt the cutting edge at a 70° to 80° angle to the stick. The cutting edge must be adapted in the same manner as you use for a tooth surface.

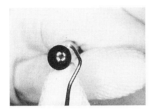

The <u>lower shank</u> of the instrument <u>should be parallel</u> (∥) to the long axis of the stick.

16. **Test for sharpness.** Activate several working strokes over the surface of the test stick. If the cutting edge is sharp, it will grasp the test stick.

It is possible for one section of the cutting edge to be sharp while other sections are dull.

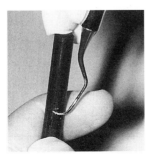

<u>Test all three sections of the cutting edge.</u> A dull section will slide over the surface of the test stick. Use a few more sharpening strokes on any section of the cutting edge that is still dull.

17. **If sharpening a sickle scaler or universal curet:**	17. **If sharpening a double-ended area-specific curet:**
• Turn the working end so that the tip or toe is facing away from you. • Repeat Steps 1 through 16 to sharpen the second cutting edge on the same working end. • When finished, sharpen both cutting edges on the other end of a double-ended instrument.	• Flip the instrument over and position the opposite working end for sharpening. For example, if you just sharpened the lower edge of a Gracey 11, flip the instrument and position the lower edge of the Gracey 12 for sharpening. • Follow Steps 1 through 17 to sharpen the opposite working end of the instrument.

SHARPENING PERIODONTAL FILES

Equipment: A metal file, called a tanged file, is used to sharpen a periodontal file.

Technique:
1. Stabilize your hand on a counter top.
2. Lay the tanged file in a horizontal position against the first cutting edge. Move the file back and forth across the cutting edge.
3. Repeat the same procedure for each of the file's cutting edges.
4. Use a plastic test stick to evaluate the sharpness of the instrument.

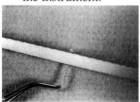

A tanged file is used to sharpen periodontal files.

Section 4:

Sharpening Aids

Photocopy this page and use it for a quick reference guide when sharpening instruments. Place the photocopied summary sheet in a plastic page protector for longer use.

SHARPENING SUMMARY SHEET

1. Hold the instrument in non-dominant hand; rest your hand and arm on a stable work surface.
2. Lubricate the stone.
3. Position the working end:

   Right-Handed Clinician

   Sickle Scalers and Universal Curets:

   - Tip/Toe toward you for right cutting edge
   - Tip/Toe away for the second cutting edge

   For Area-Specific Curets:
   - Toe toward you for ODD-numbered working ends
   - Toe away for EVEN-numbered working ends

   Left-Handed Clinician

   Sickle Scalers and Universal Curets:

   - Tip/Toe toward you for left cutting edge
   - Tip/Toe away for the second cutting edge

   For Area-Specific Curets:
   - Toe toward you for EVEN-numbered working ends
   - Toe away for ODD-numbered working ends

4. Position the face so that it is parallel (=) to the counter top.
5. Grasp the lower third of the sharpening stone in the dominant hand. Place the stone against the lateral surface.
6. Swing the lower end of the stone closer to the back of the working end until the stone meets the face at approximately a 75° angle.
7. Activate a few light strokes on the heel-third of the cutting edge. Reposition the stone to sharpen the middle-third and then the toe/tip-third of the working end.
8. For curets, turn the working end so that you are looking at the lateral surface. Make sure that the face is still parallel to the counter top. Sharpen the toe of the instrument.
9. For curets, turn the working end so that you are looking at the toe. Use semicircular strokes to round the back of the working end.
10. Use a plastic test stick to test for sharpness of each section of the cutting edge.

SHARPENING GUIDE
Right-Handed Clinicians

Photocopy this page for your use during sharpening.

Sharpening Guide for Right-Handed Clinicians

Fold the page in half along the heavy black line. Place the folded page on a counter top so that the black line is aligned with the edge of the counter.

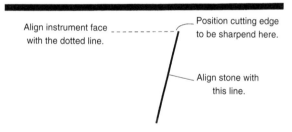

Align instrument face with the dotted line.

Position cutting edge to be sharpend here.

Align stone with this line.

Left-Handed Clinicians

Photocopy this page for your use during sharpening.

Sharpening Guide for Left-Handed Clinicians

Fold the page in half along the heavy black line. Place the folded page on a counter top so that the black line is aligned with the edge of the counter.

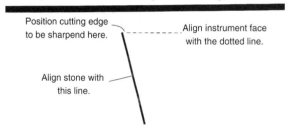

Position cutting edge to be sharpend here.

Align instrument face with the dotted line.

Align stone with this line.

DIRECTIONS FOR USE OF SHARPENING GUIDE

1. Fold the page along the heavy black line. Place it on the counter so that the heavy black line falls along the edge of the counter.

   Place a book on the top of the page to secure it to the counter or tape the page to the counter.

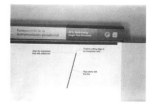

2. Grasp the instrument in your non-dominant hand; rest your hand on the counter.

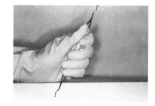

3. Align the instrument face with the fine dotted line.

   Continue with Step 4 on the next page.

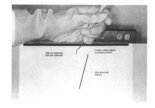

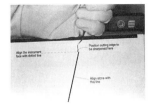

4. **Right-handed clinicians:** Keeping the face aligned with the dotted line, slide your hand over until the cutting edge to be sharpened is positioned at the far right-hand side of the dotted line.

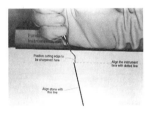

4. **Left-handed clinicians:** Keeping the face aligned with the dotted line, slide your hand over until the cutting edge to be sharpened is positioned at the far left-hand side of the dotted line.

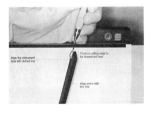

5. Align the sharpening stone with the vertical black line. This is the correct angulation for sharpening.

Section 5:

References and Suggested Readings

Balevi, B.: Engineering specifics of the periodontal curet's cutting edge [published erratum appears in J Periodontol Sep;67(9):951, 1996] J Periodontol Apr;67(4):374-8, 1996.

Bower, R.C.: An aid for sharpening periodontal instruments. Aust Dent J Aug;28(4):212-4, 1983.

Burns, S.: It's about time to get on the cutting edge. Chicago, IL: Hu-Friedy Manufacturing Company, Inc., 1995.

Claney, P.: Sharpening hand cutting instruments. Dent Assist Nov-Dec;55(6):23-4, 1986.

Cottone, J.A., Terezhalmy, G.T., Molinari, J.A.: Practical infection control in dentistry. Philadelphia, PA: Lea & Febiger, 1991.

Hoffman, L.A., Gross, K.B., Cobb, C.M., Pippin, D.J., Tira, D.E.: Assessment of curette sharpness. J Dent Hyg Oct;63(8):382-7, 1989.

Hu-Friedy® hygiene catalog & Reference guide. Chicago, IL: Hu-Friedy Manufacturing Company, Inc., 1993.

Marquam, B.: Keep eye on sharpening techniques to prevent disease transmission. RDH Aug;12(8):20-1, 23, 1992.

Marquam, B.J.: Strategies to improve instrument sharpening. Dent Hyg Jul-Aug;62(7):334-8, 1988.

Murray, G.H., Lubow, R.M., Mayhew, R.B., Summitt, J.B., Usseglio, R.J.: The effects of two sharpening methods on the strength of a periodontal scaling instrument. J Periodontol Jul;55(7):410-3, 1984.

O'Hehir, T.: New technology edges toward tools that stay sharp longer. RDH Jan;13(1):16, 1993.

Pack, A.R.: Sharpening the curette for root planing. J N Z Soc Periodontol Nov;60:10-1, 1985.

Pape, H.R. Jr., Makinen, K.K.: Verification and maintenance of dental explorer sharpness. Oper Dent Nov-Dec;19(6):221-3, 1994.

Paquette, O.E., Levin, M.P.: The sharpening of scaling instruments: I. An examination of principles. J Periodontol Mar;48(3):163-8, 1977.

Paquette, O.E., Levin, M.P.: The sharpening of scaling instruments: II. A preferred technique. J Periodontol Mar;48(3):169-72, 1977.

Parker, M.E.: Recontouring instruments to prolong life. RDH 3:44, 1983.

Rossi, R., Smukler, H.: A scanning electron microscope study comparing the effectiveness of different types of sharpening stones and curets. J Periodontol Nov;66(11):956-61, 1995.

Schulze, M.B.: Instrument sharpening—"the flat stone in motion." Dent Hyg News Summer;3(3):7, 13, 1990.

Smith, B.A., Setter, M.S., Caffesse, R.G., Bye, F.L.: The effect of sharpening stones upon curet surface roughness. Quintessence Int Sep;18(9):603-13, 1987.

Tal, H., Panno, J.M., Vaidyanathan, T.K.: Scanning electron microscope evaluation of wear of dental curettes during standardized root planing. J Periodontol Sep;56(9):532-6, 1985.

Wehmeyer, T.E.: Chairside instrument sharpening. Quintessence Int Sep;18(9):615-7, 1987.

Zimmer, S.E.: Instrument sharpening—sickle scalers and curettes. Dent Hyg Jan;52(1):21-4, 1978.

9

Dental Implants

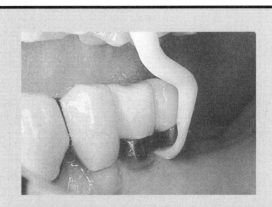

In this chapter

Section 1:

Types of Dental Implants

The two most common types of dental implants are **subperiosteal** and **endosseous** implants.

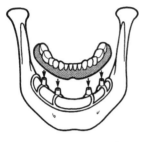

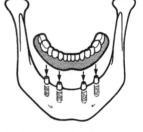

Subperiosteal implants are placed on top of the bone. The metal posts on the framework protrude through the tissue into the mouth and attach to a prosthesis. This system is used when the depth or width of the remaining bone is insufficient to accommodate endosseous implants.

Endosseous implants are placed into the bone. An abutment post protrudes through the tissue into the mouth and can support removable prosthetic overdentures, dentist-retrievable dentures, or fixed prosthetic crowns.

THE IMPLANT PROCESS

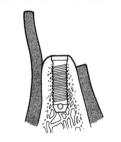

Stage 1: The First Surgery. An implant fixture is placed into the bone, and the tissue is sutured back over the top of the fixture. This fixture serves as the anchor for the dental implant. Fixture shapes include screws, cylinders, or blades.

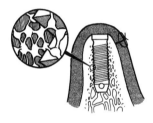

Stage 1: Osseointegration. Bone cells grow until the bone is in close contact with the surface of the implant fixture. Osseointegration occurs in 6 to 9 months in the maxilla and 3 to 6 months in the mandible.

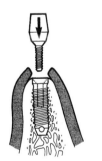

Stage 2: The Second Surgery. During the second surgery, the top of the implant fixture is exposed and a titanium abutment is attached. The titanium abutment post protrudes through the tissue into the mouth and is termed the **"transgingival abutment post."** The transgingival abutment post will allow tissue healing around the implant. The titanium abutment is extremely biocompatible and is not rejected by the body.

Stage 2: Biological Seal.
The epithelium adapts to
the titanium abutment creating a biological seal.
Peri-implant tissues are
the tissues that surround
the dental implant:

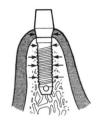

- The biological seal surrounds the transgingi-
  val abutment.
- A firm band of connec-
  tive tissue is apical to
  the biological seal; the
  connective tissue does
  not insert into the titanium as it does into
  the cementum of a nat-
  ural tooth.
- Osseointegrated bone
  surrounds the implant
  fixture.

**Stage 3: Restorative
Phase, Option 1.** In Stage
3, the abutment post is
used to connect the fixture
to a prosthesis. If the patient is fully edentulous,
one restorative option is
a removable prosthetic
overdenture. This prosthesis is similar to a traditional full denture except
it is attached in the mouth
by magnets, o-rings, or
clips. The patient should
remove the prosthesis over-
night and for cleaning.

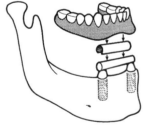

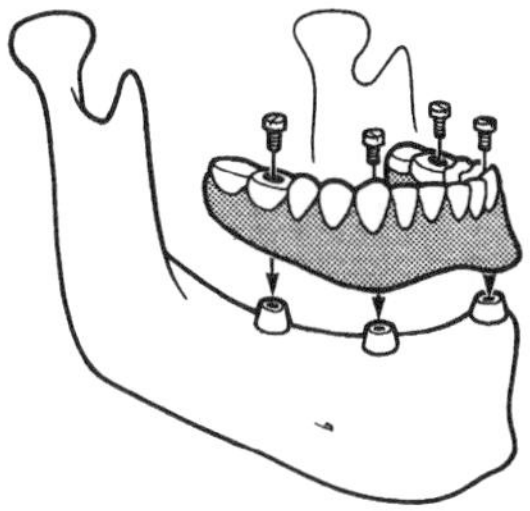

Stage 3: Restorative Phase, Option 2. A second option for the completely edentulous patient is a dentist-retrievable denture. This prosthesis is secured through the occlusal surfaces of the denture by tiny screws that attach to the top of the implant abutments. The denture is similar to a traditional fixed bridge; however, it can be removed by the restorative dentist. For this reason, the prosthesis is known as a "dentist-retrievable" or a "fixed removable" denture.

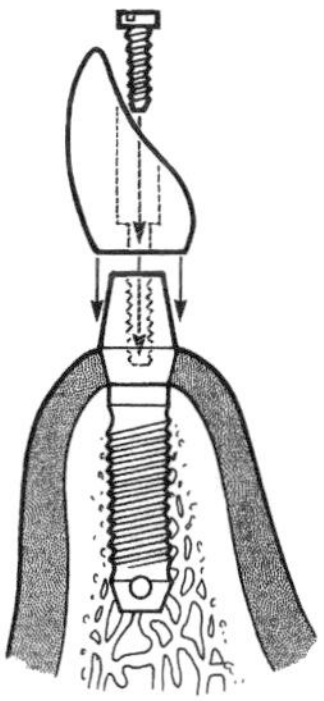

Stage 3: Restorative Phase, Option 3. A partially edentulous patient missing one or more teeth may elect to have one or more fixed prosthetic crown. A porcelain, acrylic, or composite tooth fits over the abutment. Porcelain crowns offer superior esthetics, and porcelain margins can be extended subgingivally for esthetic purposes on anterior teeth.

Section 2:

Guidelines for Debridement of Dental Implants

Special instruments are used for debridement of dental implants. The surface of the titanium abutment can be easily removed by metal instruments. Stainless steel and carbon steel instruments should not be used on dental implants. The use of ultrasonic or sonic devices with metal tips also is contraindicated with implants. Metal instruments may leave scratches on the surface of the implant that favor plaque accumulation and calculus formation. In addition, metal instruments disturb the surface coating of the implant, reducing the biocompatibility with the peri-implant tissues.

Instruments used for assessment and debridement of implant teeth should be made of a material that is softer than the implant material. Plastic instruments are most commonly used. Plastic instruments are available in a variety of designs, some of which have working ends that are similar to conventional periodontal probes, sickle scalers, and universal curets. Plastic instruments are safe for use on all types of implants without damage to the abutment surface.

Calculus is removed readily from implants because there is no interlocking or penetration of the deposit with the implant surface. Light lateral pressure with a plastic instrument is recommended; care must be taken not to scratch the surface of the implant.

A separate category of implant instruments is comprised of instruments made of plastic materials containing graphite fillers. These instruments work well on the implant superstructure (i.e., denture or prosthetic crown) but can produce scratching of certain types of abutments. For this reason, this category of implant instruments should be limited to use on the implant superstructure. Plastic instruments containing graphite fillers should not be used directly on the implant abutment.

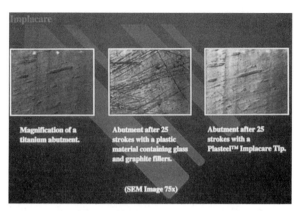

High power magnification of a titanium abutment. (SEM image 75x)

Abutment after 25 strokes with a plastic instrument containing glass or graphite fillers. (SEM image 75x)

Abutment after 25 strokes with Implacare plastic instrument. (SEM image 75x)

SEM = scanning electron microscope.
(Scanning electron microscope images courtesy of Hu-Friedy Manufacturing Company, Inc.)

SEQUENCE OF PROCEDURES FOR MAINTENANCE VISIT

1. Review of medical history
2. Review of dental history: look for history of discomfort or difficulty in function, mastication, or speaking with the dental implant
3. Soft tissue examination
4. Radiographic examination
5. Clinical examination: presence of plaque, gingival inflammation, bleeding, and implant mobility
6. Restorative integrity of implant
7. Occlusion
8. Reinforcement of patient plaque control techniques when necessary; super floss, end tufted toothbrushes, and interproximal brushes demonstrated to the patient
9. Removal of plaque and calculus with plastic instruments, tufted brushes, and irrigation with 0.12% chlorhexidine
10. Removal of dentist-retrievable prostheses by means of copings or screws once a year to ascertain gingival health and implant stability

GUIDELINES FOR DEBRIDEMENT OF IMPLANTS

- The titanium surface of the abutment is easily removed. Great care must be taken not to scratch the titanium abutment or disrupt the biological seal.
- Plastic instruments are recommended. Metal instruments and ultrasonic or sonic devices with metal tips are contraindicated.
- Instrumentation should be restricted to supragingival deposit removal.
- Strokes should be short, controlled, and activated with light pressure. Calculus does not adhere to titanium as tenaciously as on natural teeth.
- Use the basic skills of operator and patient positions, grasp, and fulcrum.
- Direction of strokes is in an oblique, vertical, or horizontal direction away from the peri-implant tissues.

Section 3:

Hand-Activated Instruments

PLASTIC INSTRUMENTS

Instrument working ends can be classified into one of four design types: (1) wrench-shaped, (2) crescent-shaped, (3) hoelike, and (4) working ends that are similar to conventional metal periodontal instruments (e.g., probe, sickle scaler, curet). It is recommended that an instrument kit contain all four of these working end design types.

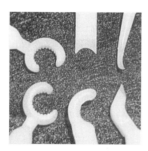

Examples of wrench-shaped, crescent-shaped, and hoelike working ends.

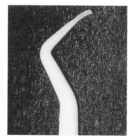

Example of universal type working end.

Brånemark System Nobelpharma Implant Instruments

Nobelpharma Plastic Instruments: From left to right, the universal, lingual, and facial instruments.

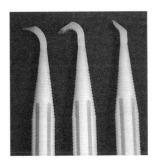

The Nobelpharma universal instrument is used for cleaning the apical portion of the prosthetic framework. Strokes should be in a facial-to-lingual direction.

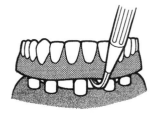

The Nobelpharma facial instrument is used to clean the facial surface of the abutment using vertical strokes.

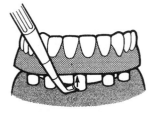

Impla-med Wiz-Stik Implant Instrument

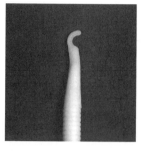

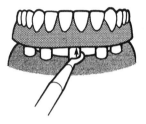

The Impla-med Wiz-Stik plastic instrument is double-ended. One end is wrench-shaped.

The Wiz-Stik wrench-shaped working end wraps around the abutment.

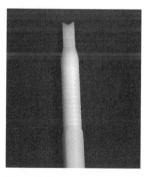

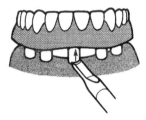

The other end of the Impla-med Wiz-Stik instrument is crescent-shaped.

Adaptation of the Wiz-Stik crescent-shaped working end to the abutment.

Hu-Friedy Implacare Implant Instruments

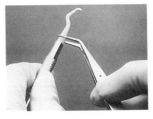

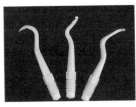

The Hu-Friedy Implacare system is comprised of a reusable sterilizable metal handle into which paired disposable plastic instrument tips are secured.

Implacare tips are available in curet- and sickle scaler–shaped paired designs.

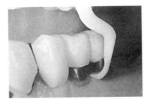

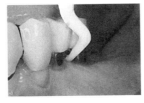

The conventional working end design of the Implacare tips is easily adapted for use around abutment posts and single implant crowns. (Courtesy of Hu-Friedy Manufacturing Company, Inc.)

Implacare tips are made of a high-grade resin that provides rigidity for calculus removal but will not damage titanium abutments or leave plastic residue on the abutment. (Courtesy of Hu-Friedy Manufacturing Company, Inc.)

Implant-Prophy+ Plastic Instruments

Implant-Prophy+ plastic instruments are made of a hard high-performance polymer plastic. These instruments are relatively new on the market and may be purchased from Advanced Implant Technologies, Inc., 8920 Wilshire Blvd., Suite 316, Beverly Hills, California 90211; Phone number: 1-800-876-4620. Implant-Prophy+ instruments duplicate the working ends and shanks of traditional steel instruments. Instruments may be reused and have good durability and the working ends can be sharpened.

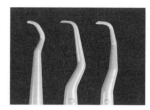

Implant-Prophy+ plastic instruments are available in Columbia 13/14U and Gracey 5/6, 11/12, and 13/14 designs. A small raised dome on the shanks of the Gracey instruments provides the clinician with a visual and tactile reference for locating the cutting edge on each working end.

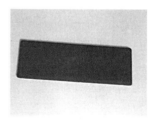

The Implant-Prophy+ instrument sharpening stone is an extra-fine grit synthetic sapphire/ceramic sharpening stone that is designed for the Implant-Prophy+ plastic instruments. The stone can be sterilized by autoclaving.

Premier Implant Instruments

The Premier Implant instrument is made of a plastic material containing graphite fillers. This instrument has a working end design similar to that of the 4R/4L curette. Plastic instruments containing glass or graphite fillers are more likely to scratch titanium abutments than are plastic instruments containing no glass or graphite fillers. These instruments work well for direct use on the prosthetic crowns or dentures attached to the abutment. Direct use on the titanium abutment could scratch the abutment surface.

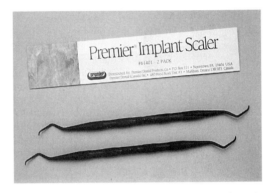

The Premier Implant instrument is made of a plastic material containing graphite fillers. (Courtesy of Premier Dental Products.)

MAINTENANCE OF PLASTIC INSTRUMENTS

Nobelpharma Implant	Can be used and autoclaved up to five times
Impla-med Wiz-Stik Implant	Are autoclavable
Hu-Friedy Implacare Implant	Handle sterilizable by autoclave or dry heat Tips sterilizable and disposable
Implant Prophy+	Are autoclavable
Premier Implant	Can be sterilized up to 140°

Section 4:

Sonic Implant Maintenance

Sonic instruments using specialized tips can be used to debride plaque and calculus from the abutments, dentures, and crowns of titanium implants. **It is important to note that metal ultrasonic or sonic tips should never be used on implant abutments or superstructures.**

USE OF SPECIAL TIPS WITH A SONIC INSTRUMENT

Example: Midwest SofTip Disposable Prophy Tips

Specialized SofTip disposable prophy tips are covered with a specially designed plastic sleeve suitable for regular maintenance of titanium implants.

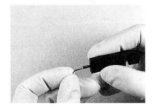

These specialized tips can be used with the midwest Quixonic sonic scaler or the Star Dental Titan-S sonic scaler handpiece.

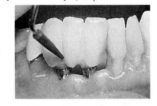

Place a disposable plastic tip in the depression of a sterilized metal holder. Insert the plastic tip onto a sterilized metal shank insert.

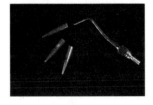

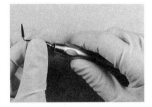

Attach insert to sterilized sonic handpiece.

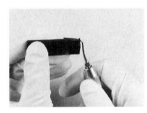

Sterilized metal holder is used to change plastic tips during treatment.

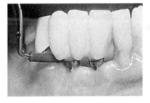

Adjust the water flow to obtain a fine spray. Adapt the tip and use light pressure as you activate strokes with a sweeping circular motion.

SofTip tips can be used to debride plaque and calculus from around implant crowns, dentist-retrievable dentures, and fixtures for removable prosthetic overdentures.

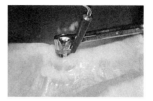

At the completion of the appointment, remove the metal shank insert from handpiece.

Dispose of plastic tip. Autoclave metal shank insert, metal holder, and sonic handpiece.

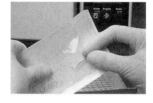

Section 5:

References and Suggested Readings

Allen, P.F., McMillan, A.S., Smith, D.G.: Complications and maintenance requirements of implant-supported prostheses provided in a UK dental hospital. Br Dent J Apr 26;182(8):298-302, 1997.

Augthun, M., Conrads, G.: Microbial findings of deep peri-implant bone defects. Int J Oral Maxillofac Implants Jan-Feb;12(1):106-12, 1997.

Boerrigter, E.M., van Oort, R.P., Raghoebar, G.M., Stegenga, B., Schoen, P.J., Boering, G.: A controlled clinical trial of implant-retained mandibular overdentures: clinical aspects. J Oral Rehabil Mar;24(3):182-90, 1997.

Bower, R.C.: Peri-implantitis. Ann R Australas Coll Dent Surg Apr;13:48-57, 1996.

Buser, D.A., Tonetti, M.: Clinical trials on implants in regenerated bone. Ann Periodontol Mar;2(1):329-42, 1997.

Cochran, D.L., Hermann, J.S., Schenk, R.K., Higginbottom, F.L., Buser, D.: Biologic width around titanium implants. A histometric analysis of the implanto-gingival junction around unloaded and loaded nonsubmerged implants in the canine mandible. J Periodontol Feb;68(2):186-98, 1997.

Danser, M.M., van Winkelhoff, A.J., van der Velden, U.: Periodontal bacteria colonizing oral mucous membranes in edentulous patients wearing dental implants. J Periodontol Mar;68(3):209-16, 1997.

Eckert, S.E., Parein, A., Myshin, H.L., Padilla, J.L.: Validation of dental implant systems through a review of literature supplied by system manufacturers. J Prosthet Dent Mar;77(3):271-9, 1997.

Grondahl, K., Lekholm, U.: The predictive value of radiographic diagnosis of implant instability. Int J Oral Maxillofac Implants Jan-Feb;12(1):59-64, 1997.

Guckes, A.D., McCarthy, G.R., Brahim, J.: Use of endosseous implants in a 3-year-old child with ectodermal dysplasia: case report and 5-year follow-up. Pediatr Dent May-Jun;19(4):282-5, 1997.

Hallmon, W.W., Waldrop, T.C., Meffert, R.M., Wade, B.W.: A comparative study of the effects of metallic, nonmetallic, and sonic instrumentation on titanium abutment surfaces. Int J Oral Maxillofac Implants Jan-Feb;11(1):96-100, 1996.

Implants Advance into the 21st Century. The International Congress of Oral Implantologists World Congress XVI in Association with the Sociedad Espanola de Implantes. Madrid, Spain: October 18-20, 1996. Abstracts. Implant Dent Spring;6(1):38-43, 1997.

Kuempel, D.R., Johnson, G.K., Zaharias, R.S., Keller, J.C.: The effects of scaling procedures on epithelial cell growth on titanium surfaces. J Periodontol Mar;66(3):228-34, 1995.

Kwakman, J.M., Van Waas, M.A., Hagens, M., Voorsmit, R.A.: Bone changes in patients with transmandibular implants. J Oral Maxillofac Surg Jan;55(1):15-8; discussion 18-9, 1997.

Liljenberg, B., Gualini, F., Berglundh, T., Tonetti, M., Lindhe, J.: Composition of plaque-associated lesions in the gingiva and the peri-implant mucosa in partially edentulous subjects. J Clin Periodontol Feb;24(2):119-23, 1997.

Mattes, S., Ulrich, R., Muhlbradt, L.: Detection times of natural teeth and endosseous implants revealed by the method of reaction time. Int J Oral Maxillofac Implants May-Jun;12(3):399-402, 1997.

Meffert, R.M.: Periodontitis vs. peri-implantitis: the same disease? The same treatment? Crit Rev Oral Biol Med 7(3):278-91, 1996.

Meschenmoser, A., d'Hoedt, B., Meyle, J., Elssner, G., Korn, D., Hammerle, H., Schulte, W.: Effects of various hygiene procedures on the surface characteristics of titanium abutments. J Periodontol Mar;67(3):229-35, 1996.

Rimondini, L., Fare, S., Brambilla, E., Felloni, A., Consonni, C., Brossa, F., Carrassi, A.: The effect of surface roughness on early in vivo plaque colonization on titanium. J Periodontol Jun;68(6):556-62, 1997.

Salcetti, J.M., Moriarty, J.D., Cooper, L.F., Smith, F.W., Collins, J.G., Socransky, S.S., Offenbacher, S.: The clinical, microbial, and host response characteristics of the failing implant. Int J Oral Maxillofac Implants Jan-Feb;12(1):32-42, 1997.

Teixeira, E.R., Sato, Y., Akagawa, Y., Kimoto, T.: Correlation between mucosal inflammation and marginal bone loss around hydroxyapatite-coated implants: a 3-year cross-sectional study. Int J Oral Maxillofac Implants Jan-Feb;12(1):74-81, 1997.

10

Polishing Procedures for Extrinsic Stain Removal

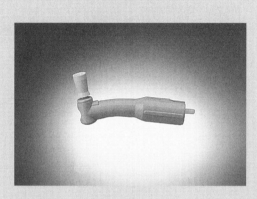

In this chapter

Section 1:

Treatment Paradigms: Polishing for Stain Removal

Polishing is the process of removing extrinsic stains from enamel surfaces of teeth for cosmetic purposes. Most commonly, polishing is accomplished by applying an abrasive paste with a rubber cup to tooth surfaces. For many years, polishing was a routine component of dental prophylaxis. Traditionally, after removal of calculus deposits, tooth surfaces and restorations were polished to create smooth, shiny tooth surfaces. The practice of routinely polishing the teeth came into question when research findings showed that polishing is detrimental to the tooth surface and is of little therapeutic benefit to the patient. Today, polishing is viewed as a non-essential procedure with limited application.

BENEFICIAL EFFECT

To improve the esthetic appearance of enamel tooth surfaces that present an esthetic problem

ADVERSE EFFECTS

1. **Production of aerosols and splatter.** Contaminated aerosols present a hazard to dental healthcare workers and patients. Clinicians and patients should wear protective eyewear; abrasive pastes contain chemicals that can cause a severe inflammatory response in the eye.

2. **Creation of a bacteremia** during the use of a rotating rubber cup polisher or airbrasive polisher

3. **Tooth surface abrasion.** Stain removal with an abrasive agent removes the surface layer of tooth structure where the fluoride content is the greatest and most protective.
    - Polishing the teeth for 3 minutes with pumice removes 3 to 4 micrometers of enamel. Over time, the loss of enamel can be significant.
    - Polishing may roughen or groove enamel surfaces.
    - Cementum and dentin are not as hard as enamel; therefore, these surfaces will be removed at an even faster rate than enamel.

4. **Heat production.** Care must be taken to use a wet polishing agent with minimal pressure and low speed to prevent overheating of a tooth.
    - Primary teeth have large pulp chambers that make them particularly vulnerable to heat generated by power-driven handpieces.

5. **Tissue trauma.** Abrasive paste is forced into the gingival crevice and even into the tissue itself during polishing. Some individuals have a negative tissue response to abrasive particles or chemicals in the paste, which can result in delayed tissue healing.

Changing Treatment Paradigms for Polishing

Old Paradigm	New Paradigm Based on Recent Research
1. Routine polishing of the crowns and exposed root surfaces of all teeth is indicated to create smooth, shiny tooth surfaces.	1. Polishing provides little therapeutic benefit to the patient and has numerous detrimental effects on teeth and soft tissues. Polishing should not be a routine component of dental prophylaxis.
2. Polishing all the teeth is indicated to remove dental plaque and films.	2. Thorough brushing and flossing accomplishes plaque removal as effectively as polishing, without the detrimental effects of polishing. Plaque begins to reform immediately after polishing; successful maintenance depends on effective daily plaque control by the patient. The treatment time that would have been allotted to polishing instead is spent in helping the patient master plaque control techniques.

continued

Old Paradigm	New Paradigm Based on Recent Research
3. Polishing is indicated to remove all extrinsic stains from tooth surfaces.	3. Extrinsic stains are not etiologic factors for periodontal disease. Polishing is a cosmetic procedure that is indicated only for removal of extrinsic stains on enamel surfaces that present an esthetic problem when the patient smiles. The polishing of thin enamel, cementum, or dentin surfaces is contraindicated. Stain incorporated in calculus deposits can be removed during instrumentation with sickle scalers, curets, ultrasonic, or sonic instruments.
4. Polishing is indicated before a professionally applied fluoride treatment to ensure adequate uptake of fluoride.	4. Polishing before a professionally applied fluoride treatment does NOT improve fluoride uptake.
5. Polishing of the occlusal surfaces is indicated before sealant application.	5. Plaque removal accomplished by tooth brushing with toothpaste, an explorer, and forceful rinsing with water or by air-polishing effectively prepares the occlusal surfaces for sealant placement.

CONTRAINDICATIONS FOR POLISHING

Factors Related to the Patient's Systemic Health

1. Patient who has a communicable disease that could be spread by aerosols
2. Patient who is susceptible to bacteremia (e.g., patients with damaged or abnormal heart valves, prosthetic heart valves, prosthetic joint replacements, rheumatic heart disease, congenital heart disease, or ventriculoatrial and ventriculoperitoneal shunts; patients who underwent cardiac bypass surgery within the last 6 months or who undergo dialysis)
3. Patient who has a high susceptibility to infection that can be transmitted by contaminated aerosols (e.g., patients with respiratory disease, pulmonary disease [difficulty breathing]; patients who have difficulty swallowing; patients who are debilitated, immunosuppressed, or immunocompromised)

Factors Related to Oral Conditions

1. Immediately following subgingival instrumentation, abrasive particles can become embedded in the pocket epithelium resulting in delayed tissue healing or, in some cases, a negative tissue reaction to the abrasive.
2. Irritants from the paste can enter the gingival tissue and the rotating rubber cup can traumatize the gingiva producing inflamed gingival tissue.
3. Tooth surfaces with extrinsic stain where stain is incorporated into plaque or calculus; stain can be removed during deplaquing and calculus removal.
4. Areas of thin or deficient enamel; cementum or dentin surfaces; areas of hypersensitivity
5. Caries susceptible teeth; areas of white spot demineralization; thin or deficient enamel (e.g., root caries, rampant caries, radiation caries, recurrent caries, white spots, areas of abrasion, or xerostomia)
6. Gold restorations easily can be scratched by abrasive agents. Airbrasive systems can dull amalgam and gold restorations. Use of abrasive agents on esthetic restorations should be avoided.
7. Power-driven polishers or airbrasive polishers should not be used on titanium abutments.

Section 2:

Techniques for Use

INFECTION CONTROL FOR POLISHING PROCEDURES	
Infection control	Power-driven and airbrasive polishing systems produce a high level of aerosol contamination in the dental operatory. Use of barriers, surface disinfection, protective clothing, and laminar airflow systems is recommended. Aerosol production is reduced by proper patient position (i.e., supine, head turned); pretreatment rinse with an antimicrobial solution; cupping of cheeks or lips for containment of water, saliva, and abrasive agent; and use of a high volume suction tip.
Protection of healthcare workers	Clinician should use recommended personal protection gear: gown with high neck and long sleeves, hair covering, mask, protective eyewear, face shield, and gloves. Patient should rinse with an antimicrobial solution before start of power-driven or airbrasive polishing procedure. Pretreatment with an antimicrobial rinse reduces the number of airborne microorganisms in aerosols.
Patient protection	Personal protection gear for the patient before start of power-driven or airbrasive polishing procedure includes: a plastic drape, towel or bib, protective eyewear, and hair covering. Patient should be instructed to remove contact lenses. Provide patient with tissues.

continued

| Containment of aerosols in the oral cavity | Use a disposable high-volume evacuation tip for suction with power-driven or airbrasive polishing procedure. Cup patient's lips and cheeks during treatment to contain water, saliva, and abrasive agent. |

TECHNIQUES FOR POLISHING

Patient evaluation	Determine whether polishing is needed. Polish as few enamel surfaces as possible. Never polish cementum or dentin surfaces.
Selection of polishing method	Select the method and abrasive agent that will produce the least amount of scratching or enamel removal. Use porte polisher if only a few teeth require polishing.
Abrasive paste	Use abrasive agent with fine particle size. With airbrasive system, increase the proportion of water in the sodium bicarbonate–water slurry.
Patient chair position	Position patient in a normal supine position. This position reduces aerosol production, reduces gagging, and facilitates instrumentation.
Patient head position	Head should be turned to the side, either toward or away from the clinician. This position causes the water and saliva to pool in the cheek area of the mouth, facilitating fluid evacuation.

continued

Retraction	Use fingers of the nondominant hand to hold lip or cheek in a cupped position away from the teeth. The cupped tissues will tend to keep the water, saliva, and abrasive powder inside the mouth.
Suction	A high-volume suction tip should be used to control fluids.
Application	Apply light stroke pressure; avoid heavy stroke pressure. Use slow speed with power-driven polisher.
Stroke technique	For power-driven or airbrasive polisher, keep the working end moving at all times. To remove heavy stain, keep the working end in constant motion while making light strokes over the tooth surface.

TECHNIQUES FOR CONTAINMENT OF ABRASIVE PASTE

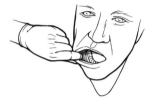

Tissue cupping for water control. Hold the cheek between the index finger and thumb, and pull out and up or down to form a cup.

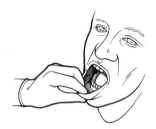

Tissue cupping for water control. Lower and upper lips can be used to help contain the water spray.

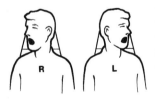

The patient's head should be turned to the right for treatment areas on the right side of the mouth, and turned to the left for treatment areas on the left side of the mouth.

AVOIDING MUSCULOSKELETAL INJURY: HANDPIECE DESIGN

The design of certain power-driven handpieces and hose attachments can contribute to the development of musculoskeletal injuries. When purchasing equipment, select an autoclavable handpiece with a hose attachment that is aligned with the long axis of the handpiece. Straight hoses place less strain on the clinician's hand and wrist than coiled-style hoses.

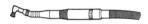

Good ergonomic design. A hose attachment that is aligned with the long axis of the handpiece places less stress on the clinician's arm, wrist, and hand.

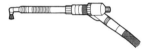

Poor ergonomic design. A hose attachment at an angle to the long axis of the handpiece exerts more pressure against the clinician's arm, wrist, and hand.

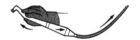

Good ergonomic design. A straight hose aligns the weight of the equipment with the long axis of the arm, wrist, and hand.

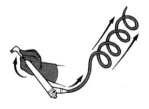

Poor ergonomic design. Coiled hose pulls against the long axis of the arm, wrist, and hand and tends to cause the clinician to flex the wrist.

Section 3:

Stain Removal with Airbrasive Polisher

The airbrasive polishing unit is an air-powered device that delivers a mixture of warm water, sodium bicarbonate powder, and air through a handpiece to the tooth surface. Airbrasive polishing can be used in the removal of stain for cosmetic purposes, sealant preparation, and preparation for bonding. Studies indicate that airbrasive polishing removes less enamel than rubber cup polishing or hand-activated curets when used for stain removal. The equipment is similar in configuration to an ultrasonic unit. Other terms used for airbrasive polishers are air polishing units, air-powered polishers, and airabrasive polishers.

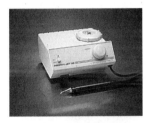

Dentsply Prophy-Jet 30 is an example of an airbrasive polishing unit. (Photograph courtesy of Dentsply/Equipment Division.)

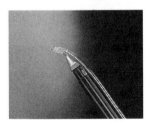

The Dentsply JetShield aerosol reduction device uses the suction from your saliva ejector system to reduce aerosols by capturing and evacuating spray. The JetShield slips over the sterilized nozzle and is disposable. (Photograph courtesy of Dentsply/Equipment Division.)

CONTRAINDICATIONS FOR USE

1. Any condition listed in the "Contraindications for Polishing" table on page 419.
2. A restricted sodium diet, including patient with controlled hypertension
3. Exposed cementum or dentin
4. Inflamed gingival tissues
5. Composite restorations

OPERATION OF THE AIRBRASIVE POLISHER

Example: Dentsply/Cavitron Prophy-Jet and Cavitron-Jet
Start of Day

1. Place airbrasive unit on a operatory counter or cart so that it is in easy reach.
2. Plug unit into electric and water sources. Open water control on dental unit.
3. Flush dental unit evacuation system with water or cleaning solution for 5 to 10 minutes before the first patient, and 3 to 5 minutes between patients.
4. Insert sterilized nozzle into the handpiece.

Fill the Powder Chamber

1. Make sure that the airbrasive unit is turned OFF before filling the powder chamber.
2. Shake powder container vigorously to break up any lumps in the powder. Screw the yellow filling cap onto the powder container.

3. Pour powder into the chamber reservoir of the airbrasive unit until the powder level reaches the top of the center tube.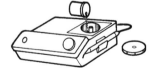

4. Remove the yellow filling cap from the powder container, and replace with the original cover.

5. Screw the powder fill cap into the powder chamber on the top of the unit. Turn the power ON, and observe the powder in the chamber. It should be visibly agitated for several seconds until the chamber is fully pressurized. If the powder agitation continues longer than a few seconds, recheck the fill cap to be sure it is securely sealed.

Technique for Use

1. Cover the unit; wrap handpiece and tubing with a barrier.

2. Connect sterilized nozzle tip and sleeve to handpiece.

3. Obtain protective gear for yourself and the patient. The patient should wear protective eyewear. Request that patient remove contact lenses, if applicable. Coat the patient's lips with petroleum jelly.

4. Position patient in a supine position; provide patient with tissues.

5. Cup the patient's lip or cheek, and use high-volume evacuation throughout the procedure to control aerosol production.

6. Position the nozzle tip 3 to 4 mm from the tooth surface, and establish the recommended angulation of the tip to the tooth surface.

Facial and lingual surfaces of anterior teeth: position nozzle tip at a 60° angle to the tooth.

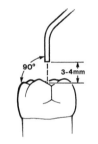

Facial and lingual surfaces of posterior teeth: position nozzle tip at an 80° angle to the tooth.

Occlusal surfaces of posterior teeth: position nozzle tip at a 90° angle to the surface.

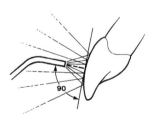

Incorrect angulation of nozzle tip. A common technique error is establishing a 90° angulation with the tooth surface. Incorrect angulation causes the slurry spray to be deflected off the tooth surface, back toward the clinician.

7. Activate the foot pedal. The foot pedal has three control positions.

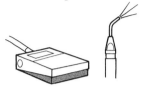

In the OFF position, the nozzle tip delivers a continuous air spray.

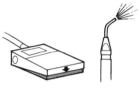

The first foot control position causes the nozzle tip to deliver only water spray for rinsing the teeth and tongue.

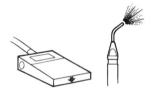

The second foot control position causes the nozzle tip to deliver the cleaning slurry.

8. Center spray on the middle-third of the surface. Polish only those surfaces that have objectionable esthetics. Use a constant circular motion, keeping the nozzle tip 3 to 4 mm from the tooth surface.

9. Clean 4 to 6 tooth surfaces, then rinse patient's mouth with water only.

After Treatment

1. Continue to wear a mask, eyewear, and face shield to protect your eyes and lungs while cleaning the equipment. Clean, and disinfect unit, hose, and handpiece.

2. Remove nozzle from handpiece sheath. Clean the nozzle tip with the wire cleaning tool. Remove wire, and use an air syringe to blow any residual powder from the tip.
3. Autoclave the nozzle and handpiece sheath. If the sheath to your unit cannot be autoclaved, wrap it in 4 X 4 gauze squares dampened with chemical disinfectant solution and set aside for 20 minutes.
4. Switch OFF the power, and remove the powder chamber from the cabinet. Use a high volume evacuator to suction any residual powder from the chamber.
5. Hold the empty end of the powder chamber away from you, turn the unit ON and OFF to clear the powder bowl.
6. Close the in-line water shut-off valve.
7. Replace the cap and bowl, and activate the unit to clear the handpiece tubing of any residual powder.

Monthly Pinch Tube Maintenance

To minimize the possibility of the red pinch tube becoming flattened, it should be repositioned monthly.

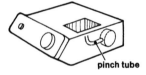

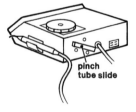

Pinch tube maintenance for Prophy-Jet model. With the power ON and the foot control in the second position, move the pinch tube slide on the back of the cabinet to the right or left.

Pinch tube maintenance for Cavitron-Jet model. With the power ON and the foot control in the second position, push the tubing into the cylinder one quarter inch.

Section 4:

References and Suggested Readings

American Dental Hygienists' Association: Position on polishing procedures. Access, Am Dent Hyg Assoc Aug;11(7), 29-31, 1997.

Barnes, C.M., Anderson, N.A., Michalek, S.M., Russell, C.M.: Effectiveness of sealed dental prophylaxis angles inoculated with Bacillus stearothermophilus in preventing leakage. J Clin Dent 5(2):35-7, 1994.

Barnes, C.M., Fleming, L.S., Mueninghoff, L.A.: SEM evaluation of the in-vitro effects of an air-abrasive system on various implant surfaces. Int J Oral Maxillofac Implants Winter;6(4):463-9, 1991.

Barnes, C.M., Fleming, L.S., Russel, C.M.: An in-vitro comparison of commercially available disposable prophylaxis angles. J Dent Hyg Nov-Dec;65:438, 1991.

Barnes, C.M., Russell, C.M., Gerbo, L.R., et al..: Effects of air-powder system on orthodontically bracketed and banded teeth. Am J Ortho Dentofacial Orthopedics, Jan;97(1):74-81, 1990.

Basu, M.K., Browne, R.M., Potts, A.J., Harrington, J.M.: A survey of aerosol-related symptoms in dental hygienists. J Soc Occup Med Spring-Summer;38(1-2):23-5, 1988.

Bay, N.L., Overman, P.R., Krust-Bray, K., Cobb, C., Gross, K.B.W.: Effectiveness of antimicrobial mouth rinses on aerosols produced by an air polisher. J Dent Hyg Sept-Oct;67:312, 1993.

Bester, S.P., de Wet, F.A., Nel, J.C., Driessen, C.H.: The effect of airborne particle abrasion on the dentin smear layer and dentin: an in vitro investigation. Int J Prosthodont Jan-Feb;8(1):46-50, 1995.

Biller, I.R., Hunter, E.L., Featherstone, M.J., Silverstone, L.M.: Enamel loss during a prophylaxis polish in vitro. J Int Assoc Dent Child Jun;11(1):7-12, 1980.

Brown, D.M.: A scientific foundation for the clinical use of air polishing systems. Part II: Technique. J Pract Hyg Nov-Dec;4(6), 14-9, 1995.

Dean, M.C., Barnes, D.M., Blank, L.W.: A comparison of two prophylaxis angles: disposable and autoclavable. J Am Dent Assoc Apr;128(4):444-7, 1997.

Dentsply Cavitron: Instructional manual Dentsply/Cavitron Prophy Jet C-300, dental prophylaxis unit. York, PA: Dentsply International.

De Leo, A.A.: The incidence of bacteremia following oral prophylaxis on pediatric patients. Oral Surgery 37:36, 1974.

Donnan, M.F., Ball, I.A.: A double-blind clinical trial to determine the importance of pumice prophylaxis on fissure sealant retention. Br Dent J Oct 22;165(8):283-6, 1988.

Gerbo, L.R., Lacefield, W.R., Barnes, C.M., Russell, C.M.: Enamel roughness after air-powder polishing. Am J Dent Apr;6(2):96-8, 1993.

Gerbo, L.R., Barnes, C.M., Leinfelder, K.F.: Applications of the air-powder polisher in clinical orthodontics. Am J Orthod Dentofacial Orthop Jan;103(1):71-3, 1993.

Gragg, P.P., Young, J.M., Cottone, J.A.: Handpiece sterilization: establishing an office protocol. Gen Dent Sep-Oct;41(5):396-9, 1993.

Koka, S., Han, J., Razzoog, M.E., Bloem, T.J.: The effects of two air-powder abrasive prophylaxis systems on the surface of machined titanium: a pilot study. Implant Dent Winter;1(4):259-65, 1992.

Logothetis, D.D., Martinez-Welles, J.M.: Reducing bacterial aerosol contamination with a chlorhexidine gluconate. J Am Dent Assoc Dec;126(12):1634-9, 1995.

Logothetis, D.D., Gross, K.B., Eberhart, A., Drisko, C.: Bacterial airborne contamination with an air-polishing device. Gen Dent Nov-Dec;36(6):496-9, 1988.

Miller, R.L.: Characteristics of blood-containing aerosols generated by common powered dental instruments. Am Ind Hyg Assoc J Jul;56(7):670-6, 1995.

Molinari, J.A.: Face masks: effective personal protection. Compend Contin Educ Dent Sep;17(9):818-21, 1996.

Nathoo, S.A.: The chemistry and mechanisms of extrinsic and intrinsic discoloration. J Am Dent Assoc Apr;128 Suppl:6S-10S, 1997

Nunn, P.J.: "Selective polishing"—time for a change. Access, Am Dental Hygien Assoc Jan;11(1), 40-2, 1997.

Rawson, R.D., Nelson, B.N., Jewell, B.D., Jewell, C.C.: Alkalosis as a potential complication of air polishing systems: A pilot study. Dent Hyg Nov;59(11):500-3, 1985.

Ripa, L.W.: Need for prior tooth cleaning when performing a professional topical fluoride application: review and recommendations for change. J Am Dent Assoc Aug;109(2):281-5, 1984.

Setz, J., Heeg, P.: Disinfection of dental pumice. J Prosthet Dent Oct;76(4):448-50, 1996.

Swanson, S.J., Tobian, M.L.: Facts about aerosols. Access Am Dent Hy Assoc Jan;10(1), 42-4, 1996.

Wilkins, E.M.: Removal of extrinsic dental stains "Selective Polishing." Canadian Dent Hyg 20:59, 1986.

Index